# The FASTER WAY TO FAT LOSS AFTER 40

Proven Methods for Balancing **Hormones** Naturally, Boosting **Metabolism**, and Achieving Sustainable **Weight Loss** for Vibrant Health & Longevity

## Cynthia A. Ray, MPH, RDN

# DEDICATION

This book is dedicated to my husband, Corey, and our three children, Cooper, Camble, and Charlotte. Their unwavering support and love have been the driving force behind my God-given desire to minister wellness education over all these years. They have made our life such a beautiful adventure together.

# Fat Loss Over 40 Group

Starting your journey with Faster Way to Fat Loss After 40?

You don't have to do it alone.

If you'd love support, guidance, and real accountability as you go through the book, I'd like to invite you to join our **Faster Way to Fat Loss After 40 Collective.**

How to Be Fit, Fabulous, and Fierce After 40

You'll get weekly trainings, group coaching with Cynthia, guest speakers, step-by-step guidance through the book, and support in our private chat, so you're never doing it alone.

This is a monthly membership; you can join anytime and stay as long as you need, then step away or jump back in whenever you want a boost.

Visit the link below to learn more: https://bit.ly/Over40Collective

# Foreword

It is my profound pleasure to introduce **"The Faster Way to Fat Loss After 40,"** a revolutionary guide authored by the visionary Cynthia A. Ray. Cynthia's holistic approach to wellness is nothing short of transformative. As a holistic and wellness specialist, I wholeheartedly endorse Cynthia's methodology, which harmonizes perfectly with the principles I advocate: embracing whole-person health as the cornerstone of true well-being.

**"Fat Loss After 40"** is not just a book but a journey that begins with God. Then, it allows God to powerfully cast a vision that will challenge and change the old beliefs that have constrained you. Cynthia's approach resonates deeply with me, for it echoes my belief as a Holistic and Wellness Specialist that we are the best custodians of our health, empowered to advocate and drive significant change by embracing knowledge and expertise. Knowledge is power.

As you progress through the book, each chapter builds on the last, from embarking on an in-depth health journey. Cynthia skillfully guides you through sophisticated nutrition and fasting strategies to enhance metabolic function and sustainable weight loss without the tyranny of calorie counting.

Moreover, Cynthia delves into the psychological underpinnings of a successful health transformation, focusing on mindset and the critical role of intuitive eating. Her recommended fitness routines promise to invigorate your body and soul, making wellness an outcome and a joyful process.

Although this masterpiece is aimed at people over 40, the wisdom on these pages is gold for all who are seeking higher education in wellness and health.

The holistic journey is rounded out with practical advice on hydration, the strategic use of supplements, and advanced fasting techniques, all designed to ensure that your path to health is as enriching as it is enduring.

"Fat Loss After 40" is a manifesto for anyone who seeks to reclaim their health authentically and sustainably. It teaches us that the tools for a transformative health experience are within our grasp. We need only to harness them with intention and wisdom.

Cynthia has crafted a masterful guide that is sure to inspire and equip you with the tools to become the best version of yourself. I will read this book over and over again. It has quickly become a health and wellness reference for me. Embrace this journey with an open heart and mind, and prepare to be amazed by where it takes you. Welcome to the first day of the rest of your healthier life.

Straighten Your Crown,
BLESSINGS,
Dr. Pamela Henkel
Holistic & Wellness Specialist

# Table of Contents

# Introduction

*How beautiful you are, my darling! Oh, how beautiful!*
*Song of Songs 1:15 NIV*

Imagine shedding stubborn weight, losing your bloated belly, aging in reverse, getting lean and fit, and looking at least 10-15 years younger. It can all be accomplished without sacrificing precious time with your spouse, kids, and grandkids, traveling freely, feeling beautifully sexy for your spouse or potential mate, and having the energy and vitality to show up fully for your family and God's calling on your life. This life can be yours by following the steps in the following chapters. You can also choose not to. Just know that not taking these steps will not only hold you back from your dreams but your situation will worsen exponentially over time.

Before we begin, let's be clear: aging doesn't have to equate to looking drab and out of shape. It's perfectly okay to love how you look and feel your best as you age. There's something special about seeing yourself in the mirror or a photo and genuinely liking what you see. You don't have to wait until you reach your goal weight to feel this way. *"How beautiful you are, my darling! Oh, how beautiful!" (Song of Songs 1:15).* Also, there's nothing inherently wrong with body fat. In God's wisdom, your fat cells act as storage units for toxins, excess sugars, water, and even harmful forms of estrogen — keeping these away from your vital organs. The issue comes when those storage sites get overloaded. Fat was designed as a protective mechanism, not something to abuse, but something your body can rely on when unwanted substances enter and need a safe place to go.

I want to welcome you to the beginning of an extraordinary journey created just for you. Today starts your path to a fresh, revitalized body, ageless beauty, and a brand-new chapter in this incredible season of life over 40. This program isn't a pursuit of vanity but a celebration of your inherent beauty, a reflection of the unique and precious individual you are.

On our journey together, you will experience more than a physical transformation. You will learn how your mindset and beliefs can be the key to making or breaking your transformation. Together, we will lean into the truths of God's word, breaking through barriers that have tripped you up in the past.

Throughout this transformative process, you will track your physical and mental/emotional health. This program isn't just about numbers — it's about strengthening your mind, body, and soul, nurturing your spiritual wellness, and learning to embrace change as it comes.

Your body is not a computer; you cannot input an equation or the perfect eating and exercise formula, producing the exact outcome you want every time. It ebbs and flows, adjusting according to its most immediate needs. I like to use the analogy of wellness as an onion with many layers. The outermost layer is the highest need that your body has at the given moment. As you progress through the steps of this program, you will peel back one layer at a time. Sometimes, a single action step leads to unpeeling multiple layers at once.

The first layer may result in more energy and better sleep. The second may be better joint mobility and no more bloating. The third may be weight loss; the fourth, a mindset shift, etc. Just know that weight loss isn't always the top layer, but it is more often than not. Remember to celebrate each layer, even if it is not weight loss. Your body needs to make adjustments to release excess body fat and toxins, so sit back and follow my lead.

In recent years, there's been a surge in research and scientific interest in weight loss. More healthcare professionals and scientists are studying human metabolism and discovering how our bodies burn fat for fuel. This renewed focus has brought back age-old principles, now being rediscovered for modern-day use.

These chapters might contain information that shakes up what you've always believed. New research is challenging old ways of thinking about weight loss. It's natural to want to dodge challenging moments, but staying open-minded and reading on can lead to significant transformations.

Let's explore and fully embrace the transformative potential that lies ahead. Always remember, as hard as it can be, to stay in your lane, run your race, stay focused, and avoid comparison. You're doing this to become the best version of yourself, not the best version of someone else.

Just know that during your wellness journey, you might blame yourself for not seeing immediate weight loss. Remember, the ***"wellness onion,"*** your body prioritizes its essential needs first. Here are some common self-criticisms I've heard from clients over the years that you may be able to relate to.

- "I've failed before, so I'll fail again."

- "I just don't have it in me."

- "I am a failure."

- "I'm just too old."

- "My body doesn't release weight easily anymore."

In times of hardship and confusion, I always return to the wisdom the Lord revealed. He reminds me that each day is a fresh opportunity to begin again. Take my hand, and let's get started. Your day one begins now!

I'm ready to guide you through this thoughtfully crafted 10-step plan tailored for fabulous women over 40 like you. With my experience and support, you can embark on this journey confidently, knowing that I've been in your shoes and helped many women like you.

Just know that if things get tough and you choose to go your own way and not make the changes I suggest, your desired results will remain stagnant and gradually worsen. The good news is that it doesn't have to go that way. By embracing these new daily habits, one at a time, you can improve your life and achieve the vibrant, fulfilling life you deserve.

# My Journey to Diet Freedom

It's been quite a journey from where I began to where I am now. About 27 years ago, I overcame my battles with anorexia, bulimia, and exercise addiction. Today, I am happy to say that I'm not just free from those struggles, but more importantly, my heart is liberated from the constant blame and shame I had placed on myself regarding my body weight, shape, and the food choices I made.

For the past 25 years, I have been a registered dietitian, taught and lived a clean, balanced lifestyle: three meals, two snacks a day, listening to hunger cues, and steering clear of calorie counting. It worked like a charm until I hit 45. Suddenly, the same routine wasn't giving me the results it used to.

In the summer of 2022, I decided it was time for a change. I invested in a one-on-one weight loss course and embraced a calorie-restricted meal plan, which I had never done since my recovery. I continued my regular workouts and monitored my weight weekly for my coach. Little did I know this journey would challenge my beliefs and habits in more ways than one.

It had been years since my eating disorders recovery program, and I haven't stepped on a scale since. Fearful yet determined, I took that scale plunge before the program started. I've been afraid of facing my weight for fear of falling back into the scale trap again. Surprisingly, the numbers didn't align with my expectations—20 pounds more than I thought. Weekly photos exposed layers of body fat that seemed to have sneaked up on me. I was confused and not sure if I should just embrace where my body was or use it as a wake-up call to change my eating habits. This reality check was just what I needed.

Unfortunately, following the meal plan left me hungry, tired, and wrestling with sleepless nights and headaches. Despite the agony, I achieved my weight loss goal, but it was a fleeting victory. Although I continued to eat healthfully and exercise regularly, the pounds crept back gradually.

A year later, after the success of my first book, **"The 21-Day Sugar Detox,"** I sensed my readers desiring more. They wanted to continue their progress beyond the initial 21 days. That's when I embarked on a new journey, diving into research and prayers for wisdom to uncover ways to help women over 40 lose weight.

A little over a year ago, during my morning prayer time, the Lord reminded me of ***"fasting."*** I had heard the phrase at church, Bible study, and from friends, but I wanted nothing to do with it. For years, I had been teaching women with eating disorders and chronic dieters how to stop starving themselves and break up with dieting. Although I was apprehensive, I was obedient to start looking into it.

Following the promising research I read, I experimented with intermittent fasting for six weeks—a 16-hour fast with an eight-hour eating window. Morning hunger gave way to a revelation: Instead of eating, I enjoyed morning coffee, tea, a good workout, and water, which became an easy way to delay my first meal until lunchtime. The result? Productive mornings, a boost of energy, a clearer mind, and fantastic fasted workouts.

Gradually, the magic happened over six to eight weeks; body fat melted away and was replaced by shiny skin, elevated energy, disappearing joint pain, and crystal-clear thoughts. Excited about the results, I invited my sugar detox group to join a test group for my new program. Twelve of the women joined. They experienced fat loss and a complete transformation—reversing aging, insulin resistance, improving gut health, decreasing bloating and joint pain, and correcting hormonal imbalances.

Fast-forward 12 months: I have led three more groups of new women through the program after the test group. I've witnessed continued success in breaking age-related fat loss barriers. I can confidently say that I've shed that extra layer of body fat along with them and now stand as lean and fit as I was in my 20s.

# Program Overview

Here is the groundwork for your success.

CAUTION: Avoid jumping right into the keto and fasting meal plan and skipping the first steps. All the steps are planned in this specific order to get results. Do NOT start building the house if you haven't laid the foundation.

Here is an overview of the journey we will take together.

Step 1: Cast your Vision

- Begin the journey by challenging old beliefs that have kept you stuck or led to self-sabotage.

Step 2: Challenging Beliefs

- How your thoughts and beliefs can make or break your success.

Step 3: 7-Day Liver Detox Meal Plan

- Kickstart with a focused 7-day liver detox meal plan, nourishing your body with rejuvenating foods and getting your liver ready for the benefits of fasting.

Step 4: Candida and Parasite Cleanse

- Annual candida and parasite cleanses are essential for optimal gut health. If you haven't done one in the past year, we'll complete them together before beginning fasting, laying the foundation for a healthier gut.

Step 5: Nutrition and Fasting for Weight Loss

- Tools to open your metabolism, stop counting calories, and release body fat.

Step 6: Fitness for Longevity

- A workout schedule designed to make you feel youthful and energetic, more attractive, and easily fit into your favorite outfits.

Step 7: Hydration and Supplementation

- Discover the vital importance of minerals and their role in proper hydration.
- Learn about supplements and tools to help you on your fasting journey.

Step 8: Mindful and Intuitive Eating

- Learn to practice mindful and intuitive eating, savoring each bite and focusing on choosing foods aligned with your body's needs.

Step 9: Top Four Tips for Maximizing Fasting Results

- Learn my top four methods for fasting with grace and sustainability.

Step 10: How to Be Fit, Fabulous, and Fierce Over 40 (Bringing it all together).

- You will learn to embrace lifelong sustainable habits without an all-or-nothing mindset.

This journey is going to shake things up for you. The power to thrive is right in your hands. As you dive into these pages, you'll find that change isn't just expected; it's inevitable! Let's unlock the doors to an authentically healthier you.

# Chapter 1

# The Current State of Our Health

*Do you not know that your bodies are temples of the Holy Spirit, who is in you, whom you have received from God? You are not your own; you were bought at a price. Therefore honor God with your bodies.*

*1 Corinthians 6:19-20*

Now that you've read the intro and know what's coming up, let's dive in. Ironically, despite living in the US and having so much available, we often neglect our health. In the 1960s, farmers faced pressure to boost crop production to feed the growing population. This rise in population growth led to the introduction of mass farming techniques, pesticides, GMOs, preservatives, and convenience foods, with each person in the US supplied with around 2,000 calories worth of food, way more than needed.

Our lifestyles changed with more women joining the workforce and households needing two incomes to manage expenses. Families became more disconnected, and convenience processed foods became a staple for busy lives. These foods, packed with sugar, salt, and unhealthy fats, were designed to keep us returning for more. Traditional home-cooked family dinners and bonding over meals became rare, leading to a surge in obesity rates.

Due to the widespread consumption of processed foods, Americans are experiencing an obesity epidemic. Our fast-paced, disconnected society is witnessing increased rates of diabetes and prediabetes, even among children, along with a rise in illness, weakened immune systems, digestive problems, accelerated aging, and premature death. Recent data from 2017 to 2020 shows that 41.9% of adults in the U.S. are obese, contributing to various chronic medical conditions such as type II diabetes, certain cancers, and heart disease. Additionally, many aging individuals in the US struggle with mobility and motivation. They often experience depression, loneliness, physical ailments, and pain, leading to accelerated aging and a sense of hopelessness. It's common to hear them resign themselves to aging-related limitations, such as weight gain or loss of vitality.

As you've likely observed, the Standard American Diet (SAD) has spread to other nations where traditional diets once promoted health and longevity. In countries such as China, Greece, Japan, and Costa Rica, the infiltration of American fast-food chains in urban areas, along with grocery stores stocked with processed snacks, has led to rising levels of obesity and related health issues like diabetes and accelerated aging.

It's time for the conversations within the aging population to shift from ailments, procedures, and medications to hobbies and activities, fond memories, and friendships. Let's raise a new generation of aging individuals by taking control of our health, exploring alternative medical approaches, and not blindly following every directive from doctors. Look beyond symptoms to identify the root cause of your condition and take responsibility for your healthcare decisions. Envision a vibrant future for yourself, actively engaging with loved ones, serving the Lord, and nurturing deep, lasting friendships.

## Aging Without Limits

Did you know that centenarians, those who live to 100 and beyond, often attribute their longevity to simple daily habits? They wake up with hope, find joy, eat whole foods, have a relationship with the Lord, cherish close relationships, and engage in activities they love, like gardening or walking with friends. Their quality of life, spiritual growth, and zest for life contribute to their remarkable lifespan.

One man from Greece stood out in a documentary about "Blue Zones," areas of the world with high populations of centenarians. Despite being diagnosed with heart disease in his 60s while living in the US, he defied his doctors' prognosis by living into his late nineties. Shortly after his diagnosis, he moved back to Greece, where his quality of life changed. He had close friends, family, and a gardening hobby, looking forward to each day with little to no stress. When asked about his secret, he simply said, *"I guess I just forgot to die."*

It all starts with your mindset and your "why." Let the Lord work in you; when it gets hard, draw closer to Him, and you will come out victorious. Most people fail because they don't stick to the challenging yet simple things. "Believe in yourself and all that you are. Know that something inside you is greater than any obstacle."— Christian D. Larson.

## My Epiphany

After turning 45, I noticed changes in my body: soreness, fatigue, weight gain, and muscle loss. Initially, I accepted it as part of aging. But one day, after a workout, I had an epiphany. What if I tried something different? What if I regained the strength and vitality of my 20s? That moment sparked a shift in my mindset, and I realized I could challenge aging norms and prioritize my health with God's guidance. After a year of research and implementation, I witnessed transformations in myself and others. This journey inspired me to teach women over 40 how to reclaim their vitality.

This program aims to help women 40+ shed stubborn weight, reverse aging, and get lean and fit without sacrificing their favorite foods, vacations, celebratory meals, and precious time with their spouse, kids, and grandkids. Empowering them to travel freely, be confident, feel beautiful and irresistibly attractive to their spouse, and have the energy and vitality to show up fully for their families and God's calling on their lives.

Approximately a year and a half ago, following the publication of my first book and after praying, I was inspired to create an online course as a next step for women who wanted more. After creating this, I invited the 21-Day Sugar Detox book group to participate in a test group for my new course.

I had 12 women participate. I was blessed with miraculous testimonials that the women shared with the group each week, above and beyond the weight loss that this course was created to produce. Ladies reported the loss of joint pain and inflammation, no more bloated belly, improved eye health, lowered cholesterol, corrected blood sugar, increased muscular strength of their youth, glowing skin, renewed energy, vitality, and weight loss and body shape change they had longed for.

This program is for motivated individuals eager to change and seek a healthier, more fulfilling life after 40. You are in the right place if you long to take charge of your health and wellness, not seeking temporary fixes but long-lasting solutions. Suppose you are sick of feeling trapped by outdated beliefs about aging and frustrated with the endless cycle of diets that don't bring sustainable results. You may have been fit and lean all your life and want to know how to maintain it as you age.

This program may not align with your style if you're seeking a quick fix, are struggling with your body image or disordered eating, are unwilling to put in the effort, prefer a one-size-fits-all approach, or resist new strategies. I suggest exploring alternative options. Although many start with good intentions and are highly motivated, sustaining change demands a shift in mindset and a commitment to the process.

In the upcoming chapters, I'll provide valuable insights and illustrate how these methods can work for you. Stay focused and avoid distractions, whether it's the latest weight loss trend your girlfriend is doing or social media ads making big promises for weight loss. Let's explore the steps that have helped countless women achieve vibrancy, balanced hormones, reduced bloating, improved mobility, and boosted confidence. Next, we'll delve into the program strategy.

## Chapter 2:

# Weight Loss Over 40 Framework

*For the Lord gives wisdom;*
*from his mouth come knowledge and understanding.*
*Proverbs 2:6*

**N**ow that you've gained a sense of our nation's health, learned some tips for living your best life, and tasted what this course offers, let's explore how you can apply it.

In the health and wellness world, it has long been touted that weight loss is a mere mathematical equation: eat less than your body burns. Recent research suggests body fat loss isn't solely about the traditional ***"energy in versus energy out"*** model. Instead, factors like blood sugar levels, insulin response, liver health, and meal timing play crucial roles. Focusing on these aspects has proven to be a more sustainable approach to weight management. In this book, I will teach you how to burn excess body fat with a few minor adjustments to your diet and how to time meals and naturally balance your hormones without restricting calories or excluding your favorite treats.

On our journey together, you'll discover:

Factors that may have prevented you from achieving sustainable results and how to break past them.

1.  Uncover why releasing fat is so difficult over 40 and how to achieve it.
2.  What you need to do to regain control of your health.

## Common Mistakes Women Make

Let's start with the common mistakes that may have kept you from getting results.

**Mistake #1:** Neglecting the Power of the Mind

In our weight-focused culture, women often overlook the importance of their emotions, thoughts, and actions when it comes to weight loss. Instead of fixating on numbers, focus on understanding and acknowledging your body's signals and needs. You must recognize that weight loss is more than just numbers on a scale—it's about honoring our complex beings and listening to our bodies' wisdom.

The weight loss industry often neglects the emotional and spiritual aspects of our well-being. Understanding and embracing our whole selves allows us to navigate our journey gracefully and resiliently.

**Mistake #2:** Insisting on the Same Approach and Expecting Different Results

Are you guilty of this? Sticking to the same old routine in hopes of a magical transformation, but never coming? Well, you're not alone. Most women don't know what else to do because what they used to do to lose weight isn't working anymore, so they keep doing the same things, seeing no change in hopes of getting results, aka insanity.

The truth is that our bodies are adaptive machines and respond to what we subject them to. If you have been doing something long enough, your body will adapt and resist change. Introducing a bit of ***"hormetic"*** healthy stress and shaking things up can bring a sudden breakthrough.

Weight loss science has evolved, revealing insights beyond what we knew a decade or two ago. For example, contrary to previous beliefs, staples like eggs, butter, and meat aren't the enemy of your cholesterol. Instead, you must check your liver's ability to metabolize fats for overall health to reduce blood cholesterol levels.

**Mistake #3:** Overlooking the Significance of Consistency & Stuck Embracing a Low-Fat, High-Carbohydrate Routine.

Ignoring consistency and sticking to a low-calorie, low-fat, high-carbohydrate diet can lead to weight gain. Contrary to past beliefs, scientific research doesn't support the idea that eating more frequently boosts metabolism. To promote weight loss and hormonal balance, prioritize eating *less* frequently, increasing healthy fats and protein, and reducing carbs.

Consistency is crucial for success. You can effectively lose body fat by consistently eating less often and maintaining a diet low in carbs while high in protein and healthy fats. Incorporating intermittent fasting allows your body to break down fat and gives your digestive system much-needed rest and rejuvenation.

## Are You Ready to Go?

I know how easy it can be to want to jump in when you're highly motivated and need to lose weight right now. From experience, only around 70% of those who start this program will complete it, and 30% end up missing out on achieving all of its benefits. Don't be that person who starts strong and stops a few weeks in. Strive to be the one who rises above the norm, fully receiving what you came to achieve.

As we embark on this journey, remember to listen and stay in tune with the Holy Spirit's promptings. Seek discernment in all areas of your life, whether it's a gut feeling or a profound word from the Lord that resonates with your heart. The best part is that you won't have to sacrifice your favorite meals or those delightful coffee dates with loved ones. Imagine a life where you look great and savor every moment with the ones you cherish, fostering deep connections, bonding, and engaging in meaningful conversations.

Before we begin, let me address some common fears I've heard from women: a need for more resources, uncertainty about how to change, struggle with time constraints, and fear of a lack of support or mentorship. But don't worry, I'm here for you. I'll guide you through accessing the resources you need, show you the steps of making changes, help you carve out time, and provide the support and mentorship you're looking for.

Now that you know what it will take to achieve weight loss and ageless beauty, let's dive into the next chapter. Before moving on, take a quick moment to reflect on the fabulous potential outcome you are about to experience and the life of freedom and vibrance you are about to step into.

This program comprises ten parts: casting your vision, mindset, and beliefs; liver detox; candida/parasite cleanse; fasting and ketogenic-style eating (80% of the time); fitness; intuitive and mindful eating; advanced fasting techniques; and a lifestyle of grace. It offers a complete, holistic package for achieving total-body wellness without calorie counting, long workouts, or sacrificing vacation and date-night foods! Let's begin with step one, ***"Casting Your Vision."***

# Chapter 3:

# Casting Your Vision

*Therefore we do not lose heart. Though outwardly we are wasting away, yet inwardly we are being renewed day by day. For our light and momentary troubles are achieving for us an eternal glory that far outweighs them all. So we fix our eyes not on what is seen, but on what is unseen, since what is seen is temporary, but what is unseen is eternal.*

*2 Corinthians 4:16-18*

Now that you understand what lies ahead, imagine your ideal health and wellness lifestyle. Do you envision presenting yourself confidently or hiding behind a facade? What motivates your journey—external pressures, societal norms, or a desire for perfection? Are you caught in a cycle of yo-yo dieting, chasing temporary highs with each weight loss? This chapter, ***"Casting Your Vision,"*** delves into self-exploration to unveil your authentic self.

Grab a journal to write in, and let's begin by uncovering the layers with a few questions for you to reflect on:

- Who do you want to make this change for?
- Why is making this change and feeling ageless so crucial to you?

- What remains of your identity if the significance of outward appearance is removed?
- How does Christ see you compared to how you see yourself?
- Who are you trying to impress or keep up with?
- Is your identity in Christ, or is it based on pleasing others?

God desires your success and fulfillment, offering value, contentment, and hope for your heart's desires. The choice lies in seeking true joy and satisfaction rather than chasing superficial beauty and living in fear.

While your body may not be flawless, the Lord can guide you towards greater physical well-being. You need the right ingredients—wisdom, resources, guidance, and the Holy Spirit—to lead you on this journey.

When I envision my grandparents in heaven, I don't see them as old and worn out as they were in their last days, but in their heavenly, perfected bodies. I imagine them in the prime of their lives, in their 30s and 40s, filled with energy, joy, and vitality. The Lord desires us to live our best lives with vitality and happiness. Living this way brings Him glory and allows us to answer His call and thoroughly enjoy our lives.

## Cast Your Vision

Start by reflecting and answering these questions:

What would your life look like in your dream of dreams (even if it feels unrealistic)?

_______________________________________________

_______________________________________________

_______________________________________________

_______________________________________________

_______________________________________________

_____________________________________________.

Think of someone who would be a great example of what you want your life to look like as you mature. (i.e., that mature woman you see playing pickleball, riding her bike, hiking, traveling, and enjoying activities with her grandkids and friends, or someone specific who inspires you)

_____________________________________________.

How would you show up (looks and attitude) in the world each day?

_____________________________________________.

Who will surround you?

_____________________________________________.

Where will you be?

_______________________________________________.


With what level of confidence will you show up in the world?

_______________________________________________.

What is your morning routine? Do you get up early, drink water, spend time with the Lord, and work out?


_______________________________________________

_______________________________________________.


Take a moment to ask the Lord about His vision for you. Grab a journal or piece of paper and start writing whatever comes to mind. Then, summarize it to keep it handy. You'll revisit this vision daily to remind yourself why you're following the steps outlined in this book.

Your reason for taking charge of your health is part of your vision. Your reason **_"why"_** behind your vision must be heart-centered, go beyond the superficial, and motivate you to persist with your wellness lifestyle no matter what comes your way.

Look within yourself, go beyond the surface, and pinpoint your most meaningful reasons. For example, why are you doing this? Are you doing it as an act of worship, thanking God for the body He lovingly created? Are you doing it for your children, aiming to enjoy a long life with them? Is it for your spouse, seeking the freedom to live on your terms, continue traveling, and deepen bonds as you age? Do you aspire to be a fully present, fun-loving grandmother for your grandchildren, sharing wisdom and creating lasting memories?

When determining your **"why,"** consider how it's tied to an apparent downside that pushes you to take action. Think about everyday habits like brushing your teeth, showering, or buckling up in a car. You do these things because of a solid **"why"** behind them and the consequences you would face if you didn't.

Write down your **"why"** here:

_______________________________________________

_______________________________________________

_______________________________________________

_______________________________________________.

Keep your **"why"** close to your heart and ask the Lord to remind you if you are starting to revert to your old ways.

The next chapter will explore how your beliefs might have caused self-sabotage or doubts in previous weight loss attempts. We'll use what we've learned in this chapter to understand how mindset influences how you respond to challenges.

## Chapter 4

# Challenging Beliefs and Mindset

*So I say, walk by the Spirit, and you will not gratify the desires of the flesh. For the flesh desires what is contrary to the Spirit, and the Spirit what is contrary to the flesh. They are in conflict with each other, so that you are not to do whatever you want…Those who belong to Christ Jesus have crucified the flesh with its passions and desires. Since we live by the Spirit, let us keep in step with the Spirit.*

*Galatians 5:16-17, 24-25*

Now that you've established your vision for a healthy lifestyle, let's elevate it by looking at your mindset. Your mindset, with its beliefs, plays a critical role in determining your outcome. *"Whether you think you can or think you can't, you are correct,"* Henry Ford said. This means that **you** choose your success or failure.

Taking this honest look within is crucial because it's only by recognizing and tackling these inner roadblocks that you can truly tap into your power for lasting change. Your upbringing and experiences shape your mindset, but your beliefs can be transformed to align with your goals over time.

Imagine starting a weight loss journey with optimism, but a few weeks in, doubt creeps in, deflating your confidence. You hear others' success stories yet question your abilities. Disheartened, you indulge in ***"forbidden"*** foods, leading to guilt and shame, fueling a cycle of defeat. Maybe you throw in the towel and resort to drastic measures, such as frequent med spa treatments or plastic surgery, wanting to look younger but instead looking artificial. The key is to learn to overcome negative self-talk, change from **"I can't"** to **"I will,"** and embrace the journey with renewed determination while seeking support, which will help you succeed.

A weight loss program that doesn't tackle mindset is set up for failure. To make fundamental, lasting changes, you must consider the whole package—your mind, body, soul, and spirit—they all work together. My friend and mentor, SoFeya SahRa Joseph, a spiritual psychologist and founder of i'MAGiNT LiFE, teaches us an invaluable lesson: *"Often, it feels like we are our own greatest obstacles. But by understanding our True Selves in Spirit and the mechanics of our minds, we can pave the way to the lasting success we yearn for."* SoFeya says success is a Quality of Spirit, and as such, our current state—regardless of whether we view it positively or negatively—is also a form of success.

For example, you can be successful at procrastinating a task you need to get done or at facing the task head-on and getting it done. With this realization, we can harness the same principles that brought us here to achieve our desired transformation. Let's explore how this perspective can guide us toward profound changes.

Let's examine the mechanism behind everything we do and create to understand this. That is our Mindset, or as SoFeya taught me, **the Mind Wheel**. Follow along the diagram and fill in the blanks that apply to you:

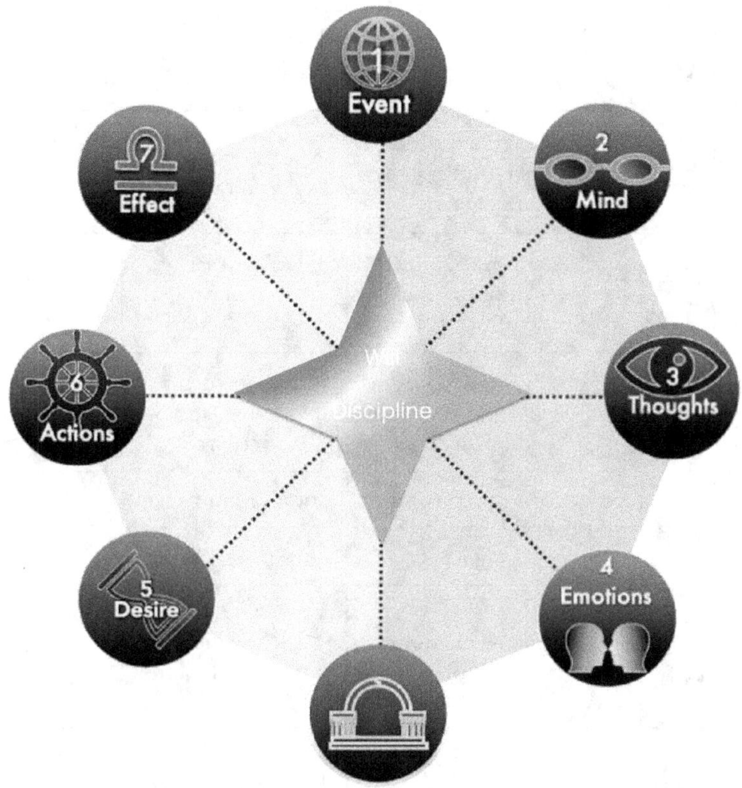


**Diagram: The Mind Wheel**

| | Mind Wheel Point | Example | Your Life (fill in your scenario) |
|---|---|---|---|
| Event | Something happens that triggers me emotionally. | Gained one pound | |
| Mind | I give meaning to the event through my mind's filters, what psychologists call "beliefs." | To be desirable and loved, I shouldn't gain any weight. | |
| Thoughts | I evaluate the event based on my beliefs and issue a judgment | This is really bad, ugly, and wrong. | |
| Emotions | Because of my judgment, I feel emotions and discomfort | Sadness, frustration, anger, shame, guilt | |
| | SoFeya calls this point the Arch-Way and is the point of **identity.** | I am unworthy, unloveable, and out of control. | |
| Desire | Because of the discomfort I feel, I desire some change | I don't want to feel so miserable. I want to feel better. | |
| Actions | I respond to my desire with action. | I eat sugar, have a glass of wine, and binge-watch Netflix to distract myself. | |
| Effect | I experience the consequence of my action | I feel like a failure. | |
| Event | Another event occurs, and the cycle repeats | I gain another pound. | |

Table: The Mind Wheel Used with permission from i'MAGiNT LiFE™. All rights reserved.

Now, let's delve deeper into the Mind Wheel. Notice how one point leads to the next, forming a continuous cycle that shapes your experience.

Notice how each (pink) point on the Wheel has a corresponding opposite (blue): your desires relate to beliefs (mind), actions to thoughts (judgments), consequences to emotions, and events to that mysterious gap that SoFeya calls the 'Arch-Way.' Here, you understand how your relationship with yourself affects your life experiences.

You may try hard to change your habits because you believe your actions cause your life circumstances. But the Mind Wheel shows us that it's not necessarily so. You might need to change the corresponding point on the Mind Wheel—your thoughts (judgments). This explains patterns called ***"self-sabotage."*** You try fixing desires and actions when you really need to change beliefs and thoughts.

When events occur, you might feel powerless to do anything about them. But what if you could change your perception and interpretation of these events? What if it wasn't "self-sabotage" but an invitation to seek more profound meaning and lessons? All of a sudden, new possibilities open, and you can choose different actions, ones that align with your true desires. This starts with examining your beliefs.

## Beliefs

Beliefs are deeply ingrained convictions about yourself, often shaped by past influences and experiences. These beliefs extend to fears, pleasures, and perceptions of the norms of aging, influencing one's views on food, body image, and capabilities. They are *"knowledge you've accepted in the past as truth."* So, beliefs act **as if** something is true and influence your future by shaping your feelings and actions in the present. That's why it is so important to question these beliefs regularly.

Another point is that most of what you consider 'knowledge' is limited based on what was known at a particular time. So, the nature of belief is limited because it was formed at a time with limited knowledge. In essence, beliefs are the lenses through which you view the world (notice the symbol used for it: glasses). Modern psychology suggests that most core beliefs are formed by age seven. At this young age, your understanding of the world is quite limited, yet as adults, you often respond to life's events unconsciously, as if you were still children.

To illustrate this point, consider this example: if you were asked to count the blue cars passing by your house for ten minutes and then questioned about the green ones afterward, you might struggle to recall them because your focus was on the blue cars. Then you might believe that green cars don't exist because you didn't see them. You form your worldview as if green cars don't exist and respond to them in kind. Ignoring green cars could create significant problems for you, and you would struggle to understand what is wrong.

That is how you grow and mature. This journey is not merely about weight management or healthy eating; it's an opportunity to consciously evolve into a better version of yourself. By establishing simple rituals to evaluate and cleanse your continual filter, you can stop recreating the past based on outdated beliefs and start creating the future you truly desire. Let's see how you can do that.

## False Beliefs

There are generally two kinds of false beliefs: **limiting** and **irrational**.

**Limiting Beliefs**—These are beliefs that constrain us in some way. They often start with phrases like *"I can't…," "I'm not good enough," "I don't deserve…,"* etc. Limiting beliefs prevent people from achieving their full potential by creating self-imposed limitations.

**Irrational Beliefs** - are beliefs that are not based on reason or facts. They are often highly exaggerated and can lead to emotional distress and unhealthy behaviors. They typically include "should" statements or catastrophic thinking, like "I should always be perfect" or "If I fail, it's a disaster." Consider the following examples of false beliefs. Can you identify which are limiting and which are irrational? Reflect on your own beliefs to add to this list.

- "Fats make me fat."
- "I have to be thin to be beautiful and acceptable."
- "Sugar is addicting; if I am around it, I can't help myself.
- "My grandmother, mom, and sister are overweight, and I am just like them."
- "Carbs make you fat."
- "I will always battle my weight."

- "I am only valuable and loved if I am thin and fit."
- "I feel so uncomfortable when someone gives me something really nice, and I have trouble fully receiving nice things and feeling like I deserve them."
- "I am a diet failure."
- "I am not athletic and can't stand exercise."
- "Gaining five to ten pounds every decade after 40 is normal."

The challenge with false beliefs is that they operate subconsciously, much like viewing the world through tinted glasses. They subtly shape your perceptions and actions without our active awareness. These beliefs run quietly in the background, unnoticed, as long as your experiences confirm them. However, when reality doesn't align with your ingrained beliefs and expectations, it disrupts this unnoticed acceptance, leading to feelings of frustration and distress.

## Breaking the Cycle

Imagine you start eating and recognize when you feel like a ***"failure or hopeless."*** Pause here. This is a perfect opportunity to hunt for a false belief, confront it, question it, and modify it to something more accurate and positive. Here, you get to interrupt your negative Mind Wheel cycle and break free from what seems like a self-sabotaging pattern. Are your thoughts helping you move forward or keeping you in shame and guilt? Catch those thoughts and replace them with truths about who you are and what you can accomplish. This is what SoFeya calls the ***"Arch-Way,"*** a point in your Mind Wheel between Emotions and Desire—a Gate out of the repetitive, unconscious cycle, an opportunity to step into your Best Self and take control over your life as a Daughter of the Most High!

Now that you've paused and identified your misbeliefs about your body, food, or weight loss, start by writing them down. It is recommended that you do this regularly.

1. **Acknowledge the belief:** Recognize and write down the false belief.

2. **Forgive yourself:**

   For example, say, "I forgive myself for buying into a misbelief as if I will always battle my weight."

3. **State the truth** (or new truth).

   "The truth is, my past doesn't define my future. I am a daughter of the most high God, loved and fully accepted by the Father. I have all the resources to treat my body accordingly, and I am free to be me."

4. **Forgive yourself for judging yourself**.

   "I forgive myself for judging myself as if I am only valuable and loved if I am thin and fit. The Truth is my body weight and fitness has nothing to do with my value."

5. **Express gratitude** for the younger self's growth through the challenging experience and appreciation for yourself for doing this work and for the valuable lesson it offered you.

6. **Ask yourself** what you want to create.

7. **Visualize Success and what** the ideal outcome looks like. Picture yourself being that already!

> "I am energetic and strong, eating healthy fats and protein with some carbs."

> "I am a master of food. I know what my body needs and enjoys food that serves its highest good."

> "I am a daughter of the Most High God, loved and fully accepted by the Father for who I am, and I grow stronger and better every day."

8. **Act As If:** Act in ways that reflect your new, healthier beliefs.

In addition, it always helps to seek guidance from the Lord, asking Him to reveal instances where negative thoughts resurface and how to shift your mindset to His truths. Scripture helps to combat negative thoughts, affirming your commitment to embracing the truth and rejecting the lies. Doing this inner work will reshape your thoughts, allowing positivity and faith to guide your mindset toward health and truth.

## Managing Stress to Lose Weight

It's worthwhile to do this work. Not only will you feel more balanced and happy, but love and peace (via a love hormone called oxytocin) will move the needle on weight and health! Your mindset and beliefs can also affect your metabolism. When stressed and oxytocin is low, your liver is caught up in the demand to metabolize the stress hormone cortisol. The result? Estrogen dominance and adrenal fatigue, increased body fat storage, chronic fatigue, muscle and joint pain, headaches—the works. Did you know that stress, often rooted in fear, is the culprit behind 98% of all diseases?

Stress doesn't stop at diseases; it also disrupts gut health. Chronic stress-related gut inflammation manifests as abdominal pain, gas, bloating, and trouble digesting food, not fun. It also disrupts the immune system, lowers serotonin and oxytocin (feel-good brain chemicals), clouds the brain, hinders memory, and accelerates aging. Daily doses of prayer, meditation, walks, or intense exercise are the keys to pumping your heart and using that excess cortisol.

Here are some strategies to manage stress and keep cortisol levels low: Engage in physical activity, prioritize morning movement, reduce or eliminate caffeine intake, consider supplements like GABA and magnesium, practice daily meditation, and incorporate regular exercise into your routine. Remember, cortisol levels are typically high upon waking up, so these practices done early can help keep them in check throughout the day.

## Train Your Brain

During my teens, I struggled with trusting food, fearing it would make me fat. This fear intensified as I entered puberty; other adult women told me that aging meant gaining weight, and I believed it! At 13, I began secretive dieting and eventually developed anorexia, bulimia, and exercise addiction in college. A year later, I sought help and spent time in an eating disorder treatment program, where I learned boundaries, self-awareness, body acceptance, and a healthier relationship with food.

Through therapy and strengthening my faith, I've begun to overcome perfectionism and now aim to help other women find similar freedom. Daily abiding in Christ through prayer and meditation, I affirm under my breath, thanking God for opportunities and growth, acknowledging unseen opportunities, finding satisfaction in my efforts, welcoming friendships, recognizing my purpose, and affirming my self-worth has kept me on track. However, it wasn't easy, and I still struggled with my self-confidence and knowing my potential for personal success. That's when I met SoFeya, and she introduced me to the Mind Wheel, a simple tool called i'MAGiNT (in the form of a drink coaster) to break free from the Mind Wheel's repetitive unconscious cycle.

Daily practice reminded me that **_"I am Successful"_** no matter what. To help me remember to affirm the truth of who I am, I have a little coaster under my water that says, **_"I am the success I want."_** every time I take a sip, I am reminded of who I am. _"No one can enter the Kingdom of God unless he is born of water and the Spirit"_ (John 3:5).

Also, remember that _"The eye is the lamp of the body. If your eyes are good, your whole body will be full of Light. But if your eyes are bad, your whole body will be full of darkness"_ (Matthew 6:22-23).

Using the i'MAGiNT coasters helps train your mind, heart, and spirit to see through a new lens, breaking through the mind wheel. It helps us clear false beliefs, release judgments about ourselves, our bodies, and our environments, and take new actions that align with our true desires.

Training your brain takes daily practice, just like any other exercise program. You must stay aware and catch yourself when you get caught in the negative Mind Wheel Cycle. Over time, you will break old thought patterns and grow and create new neural pathways, shaping fresh ways of thinking. You get a **_"Success"_** coaster for yourself by downloading it here www.yourfatlossafter40.com, and following the instructions provided.

In scripture, the Lord urges us to _"Demolish arguments and every pretension that sets itself up against the knowledge of God, and take captive every thought to make it obedient to Christ"_ (2 Corinthians 10:5). So, capture those negative thoughts aligning them with Christ's truth, and condition your mind to reflect His promises. Before the day begins, ask the Lord to go before you and remind you when you have thoughts that take you off track and pull you back down.

_"The Lord is near. Do not be anxious about anything, but in every situation, by prayer and petition, with thanksgiving, present your requests to God. And the peace of God, which transcends all understanding, will guard your hearts and your minds in Christ Jesus._

_Finally, brothers and sisters, whatever is true, whatever is noble, whatever is right, whatever is pure, whatever is lovely, whatever is admirable—if anything is excellent or praiseworthy—think about such things. Whatever you have learned or received or heard from_ *me, or seen in me—put it into practice. And the God of peace will be with you." (Philippians 4:6-9)*

And now, having planted good seeds by changing our beliefs, we are ready to adopt nutrition and fitness habits.

# Chapter 5

# Liver Detox

*Therefore, since we have these promises, dear friends, let us purify ourselves from everything that contaminates body and spirit, perfecting holiness out of reverence for God.*

*2 Corinthians 7:1*

In this chapter, we will step out of our minds and thoughts and move into our bodies, specifically our livers. But first, let me clarify the difference between three often-confused practices: fasting, cleansing, and detoxing.

While many use these terms interchangeably, they have distinct practices and purposes. First, *fasting* involves refraining from food to allow the digestive system to rest. It also includes cleansing and detoxing. *Cleansing* involves consuming specific foods or supplements to support the body's natural detoxification pathways, usually the liver and kidneys. *Detoxing* includes various methods to eliminate toxins from the body, including dietary changes, lifestyle adjustments, and alternative remedies.

## Liver Detox

Now, let's talk about detoxing your liver and why it is so important to do it annually. Most people don't realize this, but detoxing your liver is essential to weight loss. A clear liver sets the stage for efficient fat metabolism and optimal ketone production to lose excess body fat.

Your liver breaks down dietary and body fat into bi-products called ketones. Ketones circulating in your bloodstream are known for improving brain health, including mental sharpness and enhanced memory. They combat brain fog and memory loss associated with aging. Ketones are also anti-inflammatory and provide whole-body healing. However, when your liver is overwhelmed with toxins, its ability to break down fats into healing ketones limits your fat loss.

## Liver Function and Cholesterol Levels

Your liver stores carbohydrates (as glycogen), detoxifies your body, and breaks down fat. Other organs like your skin, colon, lungs, and kidneys also aid in detoxification; your liver is responsible for this process. It bears the brunt of the detox workload, processing and expelling toxins from your body. Keeping your liver free from toxins is essential for maintaining the health of its cells and ensuring it can carry out its various functions. These include breaking down fats, enhancing energy levels, promoting muscle growth, facilitating connections between brain cells, and reducing inflammation.

Most people don't know that an annual liver "spring cleaning" is a part of your wellness routine. Keeping your liver in top shape is so good for slowing down aging. It gives you a boost of energy, clear, bright white eyes, and lowers cholesterol. Your liver also metabolizes (breaks down) hormones and fats, both dietary and body stores. The metabolized fats are delivered to vital organs to assist in hormone production.

Did you know that having high cholesterol reflects the health of your liver, not the quality of your diet? Most people take medications or are on strict diets that eliminate saturated fats and emphasize soluble fiber-rich foods like oatmeal, apples, and vegetables to lower cholesterol levels. While this dietary approach does well with pulling out excess cholesterol, it doesn't address the underlying issue: a liver loaded with toxins getting in the way of your liver's job to metabolize fats.

About a month ago, my husband and I arrived in Florida for our annual snowbirding trip. Feeling bloated and tired, we wanted to reset our health. We joined my "Ageless Body Blueprint" group in their liver detox a week before they did. It worked out perfectly. Starting ahead of them, I could give them all the ins and outs of what to expect. The Sunday night before we began, I cooked a batch of sweet potatoes, quinoa, and cruciferous veggies that we could quickly reheat in the microwave for the next few days. With the food prepared, we made nutritious meals like veggie bowls and smoothies, and after just three to four days, the bloating was gone, and we felt lighter and more energized. Surprised by the delicious food, we continued the healthy eating plan. My husband even asked if we could eat this more often and add the recipes to our regular dinner rotation.

## Foods that Promote Liver Detox

Here is a list of food you can choose from during detox. These foods are great for detoxification and supporting your liver's vital functions. I created a customized liver detox meal plan for you to follow.

- **Cruciferous vegetables, such as** broccoli, cauliflower, kale, Brussels sprouts, cabbage, and bok choy, contain glucosinolates, which aid in liver detox.

- **Eggs:** Rich in choline, a nutrient that can be challenging to obtain from your diet. Choline is essential for liver cell health and fat metabolism.

- **Brazil Nuts:** Excellent sources of selenium, which enhances glutathione production and supports liver detox.

- **Ginger:** Often paired with turmeric, ginger contributes to liver detoxification. It also acts to promote gut health and reduce bloating.

- **Turmeric:** Known for its detoxifying properties, it speeds up liver detox. Combining it with ginger or black pepper enhances absorption.

- **Garlic + Onions:** These foods support glutathione production and provide powerful antibacterial benefits. For maximum benefits, consume chopped raw garlic in your salad dressing.

- **Fiber-Rich Whole Foods:** Fiber is essential for eliminating toxins. It grabs onto processed toxins in the colon, allowing for their safe removal. Fiber-rich foods include raspberries, artichokes, avocados, chia seeds, cacao nibs, flax seeds, split peas, lentils, and Brussels sprouts.

- **Coffee and tea:** These beverages are packed with antioxidants that reduce fat accumulation in the liver and the risk of liver cirrhosis. Enjoy one to two cups a day before lunch.
- **Water:** Essential for the elimination phase of liver detox, water supports sweat, urine, and bowel movements. Aim for at least half your body weight in ounces daily.
- **Almonds, Pumpkin Seeds, Bone Broth:** These foods contain glycine used to detoxify. Top your salads with almonds and pumpkin seeds, or use bone broth as the base in a detox soup.

## Foods that Inhibit Liver Detoxification

These foods/ingredients alone won't necessarily harm your liver, but using too many at a time could overwhelm it.

- Alcohol
- Fructose-rich foods include many conventional baked goods, soda, sweetened coffees, sweetened cocktails, high-fructose corn syrup, honey, jams, jellies, and anything with added sugar.
- Sucrose Rich Foods: Sucrose is the general "table sugar" in most foods containing added sugar.
- Conventional Baked Goods
- Fried Foods
- Maple Syrup

- "Fake" Sugars: Non-nutritive sweeteners like sugar alcohols, aspartame, stevia, and monk fruit can heighten sugar cravings and hunger levels in some individuals. Using these regularly won't necessarily impact your liver, but can interfere with desired results.

## 7-Day Liver Detox Meal Plan

It's time to implement my 7-Day Liver Detox meal plan. Download it at www.yourfatlossafter40.com. It includes a complete meal plan, delicious recipes, a grocery list, a frequently asked questions section, and a preparation guide. Although a liver detox may not sound appealing, you will be pleasantly surprised by how tasty the meals are.

Remember, the primary objective is to clear your liver, priming it to melt away body fat and balance your hormones. However, you might discover that you lose weight and feel much better just by completing this 7-Day Liver Detox.

## Steps to getting started:

1. Download your meal plan.
2. Print it out.
3. Take a look at the grocery list.
4. Grab what you need at the store.
5. Prepare a batch of quinoa and sweet potatoes to reheat during the week and add your toppings.
6. You can follow it exactly or make your creations based on the foods listed in the meal plan.
7. You'll love this meal plan, and it feels incredible!

Complete this in the next seven days before starting with the parasite and candida cleanse. If you encounter any hiccups in your progress, just keep moving forward and complete the seven days.

## Chapter 6

# Parasite and Candida Cleansing

*Purify me with hyssop, and I shall be clean*

*Wash me, and I shall be whiter than snow.*

*Psalm 51:7*

Congratulations on completing the liver detox! I hope it benefited you and you enjoyed the meals on the plan. Following the detox, let's spend a few days addressing intestinal parasites and candida. This step is essential if it's been over a year since your last cleanse. Along with a liver detox, ridding excess parasites and candida sets the stage for overall wellness and enhances the effectiveness of the keto and fasting lifestyle.

In the late 1800s, "deworming" was routine in the US, with children and adults undergoing it twice a year to prevent serious illnesses and complications caused by parasitic infestations. Doctors commonly used pure gum spirits of turpentine to rid infestations, a remedy also used to treat various ailments.

Many confuse "pine gum turpentine" with the "mineral turpentine" you get at a hardware store as a paint thinner. Let me clarify: Pine gum spirits of turpentine are a natural resin extracted from pine trees, traditionally used for treating various ailments, and considered an eco-friendly natural antibiotic. In contrast, mineral turpentine, derived from petroleum, is primarily used in industries like paint and cleaning and lacks the specific terpenes in gum turpentine. The key differences lie in their sources, compositions, environmental impact, and applications. Be aware of which you are buying. Go to www.yourfatlossafter40.com to find the correct one for clearing parasites and candida.

In today's world, parasites can be obtained from restaurants serving undercooked meat or poorly handled produce. Parasites and candida naturally occur in your gut, but they can overgrow if you don't give your system a good cleaning once a year. Overgrowth happens with too much sugar, antibiotics, and stress, which disrupts your gut balance and causes inflammation. Annual "spring cleaning" is essential to keeping your gut healthy.

## Parasitic Overgrowth

You can assume you have parasites if you've never done a parasite or candida cleanse. Also, if you know you have excess candida, you likely carry extra parasites.

Approximately 90% of Americans have parasites such as whipworms, tapeworms, roundworms, and toxoplasma. Getting parasites is easier than you think, even if you live a healthy lifestyle.

They can hitch a ride into your body from tap water, eating undercooked food (Including beef), touching a germy door handle, or just going barefoot in the yard. These invaders settle in the gut, where they can create tiny holes in your gut lining (leaky gut), causing a whole host of digestive problems. But that's just one part of the story.

## Common Signs of Parasitic Overgrowth:

Gut problems like these are usually the first sign:

- Bloating
- Smelly gas
- Stomach cramps
- Vomiting or nausea
- Loose stools

Parasites are active at night. They don't just harm your digestion. They can also lead to:

- Constant hunger
- Fatigue
- Unexplained weight loss
- Achy joints
- Low moods
- Worrying
- Rashes or hives
- Poor sleep
- Itchy spots around the bottom and private parts
- Frequent yeast flare-ups

- Anxiety
- Teeth grinding
- Stiff neck

## Candida Overgrowth/Infection

Can you relate to any bizarre symptoms that nobody can seem to get a handle on? Candida toxins can affect just about all cells of all organs and systems of a person's body, causing any or all of the symptoms listed below. Take a look at these symptoms and see what looks familiar. If so, there is a big chance that you may have a Candida infection.

- Alterations or disturbances of smell, taste, sight, or hearing (blurry vision, spots before the eyes, erratic vision, spots in front of the eyes (eye floaters), flashing lights off to the side of vision, redness, dryness, itching, excessive tearing, inability to tear)
- Swelling and tingling in the head
- Brain fog
- Loss of self-confidence or self-esteem
- Irritability, short fuse, impatience
- Nervousness, agitation, panic attacks.
- Poor concentration
- Dull, background headaches
- Earaches, itchy ears.
- Confusion.
- Mood swings.
- Dizziness, light-headedness.

- Inappropriate drowsiness.
- Numbness, tingling, or weakness (tongue, hands, feet)
- Poor short-term memory.
- Hyperactivity, especially in children
- Agitation
- Crying or emotional spells
- Depression, especially before a period in women
- The feeling of "cotton wool" in the head
- Feelings of being "unreal" or spacey
- Feeling drunk or intoxicated

## The Blessing of Pine Gum Spirits of Turpentine

Last fall, while my husband and I were walking by our local lake, he told me he had just gotten a text from our healthcare practitioner saying that his candida had returned. Over the years, he has faithfully followed the protocol to clear it, including a strict diet and supplements. Despite his hard work, it had returned, and he was over it. He told me that he just wanted to have the option to enjoy food and a beer here and there. At that moment, frustrated for him, I prayed for a solution. I told God right then and there how frustrated I was and demanded that He bring us the solution I knew He had.

Lo and behold, two days later, while meeting up with a new friend, Cyndi Rai, for tea, she told me about a friend who had shared pine gum spirits of turpentine with her and how it was good for killing candida. As soon as she said "candida," I stopped in my tracks. Cyndi offered to share some with me to take to my husband. She muscle-tested him for the proper dosage and had him start immediately. Intrigued by this unconventional approach, I checked out the research and found out about Dr. Jennifer Daniels through a client of mine. Dr. Daniels is a huge advocate for pine gum spirits of turpentine for many uses, including killing off candida. Following her guidance and incorporating it into his regimen, his symptoms of bloating, headaches, and fatigue had significantly improved.

However, like all powerfully effective things (such as antibiotics), you don't have to take pine gum spirits or turpentine if you don't feel comfortable. I will provide another method that takes a few more weeks but is also effective.

Here are some ways to get rid of parasites and candida:

*Pine Gum Spirits of Turpentine*

1. Follow a whole-food diet, avoid processed foods and sugars, and ensure that meat and vegetables are well-cooked. Download the "Anti-Candida Diet" meal plan (also good for parasite removal). Find the meal plan at www.yourfatlossafter40.com

2. Clearing your large and small intestines is essential before taking remedies for clearing parasites and candida. I recommend taking 1-2 tablespoons of castor oil on an empty stomach in the morning. Recommend type at www.fatlossafter40.com. If the first tablespoon doesn't take effect within eight hours, repeat the following day with two tablespoons until you have three bowel movements, ensuring your large and small intestines are clear. If you have diarrhea, that's okay.

Other than drinking castor oil, another option is to do a coffee enema two days in a row.

3. Once clear, you can begin taking pine gum spirits of turpentine while following the anti-candida diet. Take it for five days. Drop it into the middle of a small mound of ½- 1 tsp of sugar, keeping the outer edges dry, and wash it down with water. Since candida and parasites are attracted to sugar, it's used to lure them into eating the pine gum spirits, like a mouse trap. It has a black licorice flavor and is expected to burp a bit. If you don't like burping, take it at night before bed.

*Pine Gum Spirits Schedule and Dosage*

- Day One:  five drops with ½ tsp sugar
- Day Two:  ten drops with ½ tsp sugar
- Day Three: fifteen drops with one tsp of sugar.
- Days Four & Five:  ½ teaspoon pine gum spirits of turpentine with one teaspoon of sugar.

Drink at least four quarts of water per day. Pine gum spirits are a powerful natural antibiotic. *Do not exceed the recommended dosage of pine gum spirits or turpentine shared above. If you notice headaches, fatigue, or no bowel movement after two days, do an additional round or two of coffee enemas or take another dose of castor oil to help release the organisms. Your bowel is their easiest way out.

## Alternative Candida and Parasite Cleanse Method

If you do not want to use turpentine and have never cleansed candida or parasites, cleanse candida for the first 30 days, then move on to the parasite cleanse. You will use the Anti-Candida meal plan for both candida and parasite cleansing.

For the candida cleanse, use SOLARAY Yeast Cleanse capsules. If this is your first time cleansing candida, start with half the recommended dosage for the first two weeks and then build up to the full dosage.

Use Diatomaceous Earth to cleanse parasites. Recommended products can be found at my book's resource site, www.yourfatlossafter40.com.

**Parasite Cleansing Using Diatomaceous Earth (DE):**

1. Start with one tsp mixed into eight ounces of water. Drink this either one hour before a meal or two hours after a meal. The goal is to have an empty stomach.
2. Repeat this every day for ten days and slowly increase your amount of DE to two tsp if you like.
3. Once you hit ten days, take a break for seven days
4. Repeat for ten days. You may see some interesting stools being passed.

If you feel achy, tired, or have headaches, do a coffee enema a few times or take one to two tablespoons of castor oil to help your body expel the parasites more easily. To prevent these symptoms, you can do a coffee enema a few times a week or as needed to facilitate their removal from your body. With the DE, there may be some constipation, but drinking an extra glass of water after your DE drink can help with this.

Many people don't realize that getting rid of parasites and candida can reverse sugar cravings, skin rashes, abdominal bloating, making weight loss effortless. Stay on track and get excited because this is the last of the pre-work before we jump into the weight loss portion.

## Chapter 7

# Nutrition and Fasting for Fat Loss

*I praise you because I am fearfully and wonderfully made; your works are wonderful,*

*I know that full well.*

*Psalm 139:14*

**Y**ay! You have completed all the foundational tasks, and now we can finally move into the lifestyle stuff. We will focus on adjusting your diet to achieve the best weight-loss and wellness results after 40.

When you think of ***"fasting,"*** you might link it to a spiritual fast, seeking clarity from God, or intermittent fasting for weight loss. Unlike spiritual fasting, Scripture doesn't directly command fasting for physical health, although it does enhance our spiritual connection and benefit our bodies. During a podcast interview with my friend Rennie Ling, author of **"Give, Pray, Fast,"** we discussed how spiritual and fasting for health overlap. During our conversation, I realized that as our bodies enter ketosis, burning stored fat for fuel, our minds get a boost of ketones, leading to clearer thinking and a stronger connection with God. Mixing both types of fasting can give you a spiritual and physical boost. Throughout your fasting journey, invite God in and feel His love as your body heals. Then, when fasting gets tough, turn to Him for inner strength through the Holy Spirit. You will be amazed at what you can do with Him by your side.

## Fasting, the New "Old" Way to Lose Fat

Before moving into fasting, knowing who should not engage in fasting is essential. This includes those with a history of or currently struggling with eating disorders (including binge eating), type I or II diabetes (without medical supervision), if you are pregnant or breastfeeding, are under a lot of stress, or have adrenal fatigue. If you are taking medications that require food, ask your doctor if it is ok and how to structure your medication schedule.

Did you know that the long-standing advice of eating small, frequent meals to boost metabolism, which nutrition professionals and practitioners have advocated for the past 15-20 years, has never been validated in research? There is not one study that shows that eating frequently elevates metabolism. In contrast, according to an article by Healthline, ***"Studies reveal that fasting for up to 48 hours can boost metabolism by 3.6–14%."***[1] Many people believe that not eating slows it down, but we now know that is not true.

---

[1] Gunnars, Kris. "11 Myths about Fasting and Meal Frequency." *Healthline,* Healthline Media, 22 July 2019, www.healthline.com/nutrition/11-myths-fasting-and-meal-frequency.

Yes, you can and will lose body fat if you reduce your calories to less than what you expend.

However, this is not sustainable. It is only effective for short-term weight loss because your metabolism lowers to meet the calories necessary to survive. Let's say you want to lose weight and start with a 1,400-calorie diet, lose some weight, and a few weeks later, the weight loss stops. To get it going again, you move to a 1,200-calorie diet. Weight loss picks back up, and after several weeks, it stalls again. Each time calories are reduced, your metabolism lowers to meet it, and your weight stabilizes. By this point, you feel tired and hungry and have no energy for exercise. I know I went through this same thing and regained most of the weight.

## How to Sustainably Lose Body Fat

Our bodies run on two sources of energy: carbohydrates and fat. Once your body's (mainly in your liver and muscles) carbohydrate stores are depleted, either from following a ketogenic diet, intermittent fasting, or interval workouts, your metabolism switches gears from using carbohydrates to breaking down fat for fuel. We will be using a "ketogenic style" diet and fasting to reach ketosis, breaking down body fat, and losing cravings. This eating style focuses on elevating fats and protein and limiting carbohydrates. It comprises approximately 60% fats, 30% protein, and 10% carbohydrates. Conditioning your body to burn fat ("'fat adapted') and quickly switching from using carbs to using fat for energy (we call it 'metabolically flexible') helps you to sustain lifelong leanness.

Here's the overall strategy: You will stick to a ketogenic *"keto"* lifestyle 80% of the time, along with foods that promote hormone balance from the list below. The remaining 20% is your flexibility zone. This zone allows you to enjoy non-keto treats on social occasions, vacations, and holidays, or savor "dessert day" with your family without sabotaging your results. I usually recommend doing this once a week or less as the opportunity arises. It also offers the flexibility to enjoy *"estrogen and progesterone"* boosting foods during your cycle, as described below.

Side note: While you're eager to see results and stay focused on doing everything right, remember that your journey is more than achieving sustainable body fat loss. It's about cherishing moments with family and friends, creating lasting memories, and having room to enjoy special foods that are off-plan.

Adding fasting to a ketogenic diet is a potent tool for losing excess body fat. Fasting accelerates the transition into ketosis (burning fat for fuel). Eating ketogenic foods continues the fat-burning process that fasting kicked off, keeping your blood sugar stable and energy up.

An intermittent fasting lifestyle gives your digestive system a much-needed break. It's best to begin slowly with a 12-hour fasting and 12-hour eating window. Then, gradually extend fasting windows to condition your body to achieve fat-adaptation. When it is time to eat, adding lots of healthy fats, such as nuts, olive oil, avocado, and fatty fish, to your daily diet makes fasting effortless and eliminates cravings.

Fasting isn't just another trend—it has deep historical roots, recognized even by Hippocrates. Its cellular-level reset benefits have been seen in my groups, personal experiences, and private clients' lives. Fasting for fat loss is a slow but steady journey. It's not a quick fix; it's just another daily part of staying healthy, like brushing your teeth or working out. Your weight might go up and down, but will trend downward over time.

As with anything, too much of a good thing can be harmful. Avoid fasting beyond my recommended schedule, and if your cortisol levels are high, practice mindfulness daily to lower them. Excessive fasting regularly can lead to increased stress, stalled weight loss, nutrient deficiencies, accelerated aging, muscle loss, weakened immunity, cognitive decline, and hindered social life.

Here's a breakdown of the benefits of fasting based on its duration:

- **13-15 hour fast:**
    - Initiates intermittent fasting
    - Triggers growth hormone secretion (slows muscle loss), aiding in fat burning and slowing aging.
- **15-hour fast:**
    - Ketones are produced, indicating a shift from burning sugar to burning fat.
    - Ketones offer brain preservation, providing energy and improved mental clarity.
- **17-24-hour fast:**

- o Benefits include cellular repair, detox, cancer prevention, fat repair, anxiety and depression relief, and improved brain function and memory.
- **17-hour fast:**
  - o Stimulates autophagy, allowing cells to heal and repair themselves.
  - o It is beneficial for individuals with autoimmune conditions.
- **24-hour fast:**
  - o Intestinal cells reboot, increasing GABA production, relaxing the brain, and helping with anxiety.
  - o It supports gut health, prevents autoimmune disorders, and aids in weight loss.
- **36-hour fast:**
  - o Forces the body to burn glucose, insulin, and stored toxins, promoting fat loss, anti-aging, and an increase in dopamine.
- **48-hour fast:**
  - o Resets dopamine receptor sites, which is beneficial for improving happiness levels.
- **72-hour fast:**
  - o A three-day fast is suitable for those seeking a comprehensive immune system reboot.
  - o Regenerates stem cells for the immune system and promotes stem cell production for musculoskeletal injuries.

Before we go any further, let's address the elephant in the room: hunger. Feeling hungry is natural, and it's okay to experience it occasionally. However, it's important to distinguish between hunger and actual starvation. Starvation implies not having access to food, while fasting involves choosing to refrain from eating for a period of time. While fasting can have health benefits, it's not suitable for everyone, including growing children, those who have a history of eating disorders where fasting is triggering, type 1 diabetics, pregnant and nursing mothers, and those with certain medical conditions.

Contrary to popular belief, your body can handle more extended periods without food, like during a good night's sleep. The phrase **"breakfast is the most important meal of the day"** is an advertisement slogan written by James Caleb Jackson and John Harvey Kellogg to sell more cereal products. However, breakfast first thing in the morning isn't necessarily the **"most important meal of the day."** It is just one of the meals of the day. Our bodies are also able to skip breakfast. Ever notice how hunger often fades away on days when you get too busy to eat? Sometimes, it gets replaced by a slight headache or lightheadedness (which means you probably need more water). No need to panic—skipping a meal won't do any harm. It's a natural and healthy habit with many benefits, as seen in those mentioned earlier. Hunter-gatherers didn't wake up and reach for snacks; they typically had to hunt for food. Hunting in a fasted state was ideal since their minds were sharper, making hunting more successful.

Hunger is inevitable, and a growling stomach doesn't always mean you need food right now; lean into your hunger, remembering that it will come and go within 20 minutes, and you will be okay. Mineral water, black coffee, tea, and plain water help fill the fasting gap. Also, don't confuse fasting with cutting calories. Fasting just means you have a set time for eating and a set time for not eating. It doesn't mean you consume fewer calories overall than if you were eating throughout the day.

## Nutrition

Breaking your fast doesn't have to lead to an unhealthy binge, leaving you with a headache, stomachache, and fatigue. While it's normal to indulge when breaking a fast, plan ahead with *"fast-breaking foods."* When ready to break your fast, start with foods high in healthy fats, moderate in protein, and probiotic-rich, such as plain Keifer, sauerkraut, or kimchi. These foods will prevent a blood sugar spike and ensure sustained energy levels.

Make sure you're also including enough feast days. Having sufficient healthy feast days in your week can speed up your metabolism. Remember, we're teaching our bodies to be in their best metabolic shape in the presence and absence of food. On feast days, load up on nourishing foods that boost your gut health, energy, organs, and hormones. To support your hormones and nourish your body, focus on healthy fats and protein and add progesterone- and estrogen-boosting foods to your diet according to your cycle (more on that below).

## Getting Out of a Weight Loss Plateau

If you hit a weight loss plateau, switch up your fasting routine to keep your metabolism from slowing. Since your body is adaptive for survival, fasting the same way every day can slow down your metabolism over time. Mix it up by throwing in a weekly 24-hour or 36-hour fast or taking a week off of fasting, then returning to your regular fasting schedule. If you continue to feel stuck, change your diet by adding the foods that feel best for your body and continue your regular fasting schedule. Also, check in and see if you are getting in the way of yourself by focusing too much on weight loss rather than celebrating what your body has done for you. Concentrating on your weight changes can also lead to stalled progress. Consider getting rid of your scale and using your body as an indicator.

## Hormones and Fasting

Whether you're still menstruating or not, matching your fasting routine to your menstrual cycle or hormonal fluctuations is essential for hormonal health. Here are fasting guidelines based on different stages of your reproductive and post-reproductive years. (see the *"Additional Resources"* section at the back of the book for a comprehensive chart.)

## Women in Perimenopause (40-50 years of age):

Perimenopause brings hormonal shifts; fasting helps balance stress and insulin, balancing reproductive hormones.

**Days 1-10** (Day 1 is the first day you bleed): At this time, estrogen and energy are high, and you can engage in all types of fasting, including extended-length fasts. You are incorporating keto foods, including plenty of fats and protein.

**Days 11-15**: Fasting only for up to 15 hours, and "hormone feasting" foods are recommended.

**Days 16-19**: Fasting can resume with all types of fasting. The ovulation window can involve extensive fasting and a return to a ketogenic style of eating.

**Days 20** until the first day of bleeding: Progesterone levels rise, and you will need to take a break from fasting, going no longer than 13 hours without food, and eating progesterone foods (listed below) along with fats and protein. Extra supplemental magnesium glycinate over the last ten days supports progesterone and reduces cravings for chocolate and unhealthy carbohydrates. Energy tends to be low; nurture your body at this time, keeping cortisol and stress low.

## Women in Menopause (50-55 years of age):

The optimal fasting schedule includes fasting 15-18 hours five days a week, fasting 24 hours a day during the week, and one day off, including healthy feasting.

***Example schedule:***

- Sunday: Fasting day off (eat according to hunger and enjoy an off-plan food or drink)
- Monday: Extended fast 20-24+ hours.
- Tuesday-Friday: 16–18-hour fasts
- Saturday: 16-18 hour fast (enjoy a treat of off-plan food or drink)

## Post-Menopausal Women (55+ years of age):

If you are post-menopausal, you can fast freely. However, it's advised to incorporate a day off of fasting and implementing a hormone (specifically progesterone) feasting day once a week, along with plenty of opportunities to get quality protein, healthy fats, and some carbohydrates to build your body and maintain a healthy hormonal balance. You can adopt the same fasting schedule as women in their menopausal years: fasting for 15-18 hours five days a week, fasting 24+ hours once a week, and allowing yourself one day off for" hormone **feasting."**

In your postmenopausal years, another option is to fast according to the lunar cycle (phases of the moon) to get your hormones back in balance. God designed your bodies to align with nature's cycles, including the moon's phases. However, misalignment happens because most of your life is spent under blue lights and a small percentage under the sun's red light. Another reason why getting outside is so important to your health.

Let's talk about how to fast with the lunar cycle—starting with the new moon as your day one. You can Google the moon phase on a calendar and start tracking.

- Days 1-5: fast for 15 hours
- Days 6-10: fast for 17+ hours
- Days 11-15: fast for 15 hours
- Days 16-19: fast for 17+ hours
- Day 20-30: fast 16 hours max

## Hormone Building Foods

Incorporating specific foods into your diet to support hormones effectively reverses symptoms of hormonal imbalances. Focus on foods that contain nutrients essential for progesterone and estrogen production.

## Progesterone Foods

Suppose you are peri-menopausal and still have an active menstrual cycle or are following the lunar cycle; progesterone-building foods should be eaten from day 20, the first day of bleeding, or the next new moon while taking a break from fasting to support progesterone.

## Foods that support healthy progesterone:

- Bananas
- Beets
- Black beans, kidney beans, and chickpeas
- Broccoli
- Brussels sprouts
- Butternut squash, acorn squash, honey nut squash, and spaghetti squash
- Cauliflower
- Grapefruit
- Lemons
- Mangoes
- Oranges
- Papaya

- Sunflower seeds, sesame seeds, chia seeds, and flax seeds
- Sweet potatoes, yams, and red potatoes
- Turnips

## Estrogen Foods

Consider adding phytoestrogen-rich foods such as flaxseeds and legumes to boost estrogen levels. These plant-based compounds mimic estrogen's action in the body. Estrogen prefers low blood sugar and insulin levels, favoring salads over sandwiches, specifically foods rich in good fats, especially those naturally high in cholesterol. The good news is that certain foods can restore estrogen and reduce your menopause belly. During perimenopause, estrogen-building foods should be eaten from days 1-10 and 16-19, where you can do all fasting durations.

## Foods that support estrogen:

- Almonds, cashews, Brazil nuts, pine nuts, walnuts
- Avocados
- Blueberries, strawberries, and cranberries
- Broccoli
- Cabbage
- Cauliflower
- Chickpeas, lima beans, kidney beans, mung beans, pinto beans, black-eyed peas, lentils
- Fennel
- Olive oil and sesame seed oil

- Onion
- Organic soybeans
- Pumpkin seeds, sunflower seeds, sesame seeds
- Spinach
- Zucchini

## Put it into practice:

For the first few weeks of fasting, just do a 12-14-hour fast daily (e.g., 7 pm-7 am/9 am). After that, test the waters, stretching it a bit more by moving regular 16- and 18-hour(ex:7pm-11 am/1 pm) fasts here and there. Once you are more experienced and have strengthened your **"fasting muscle,"** go for five days a week of intermittent fasting (16-18 hours), one day of 24-hour fasting, and one day of no fasting but healthy feasting.

When you begin doing extended fasts or are new to fasting, you may feel low energy, blood sugar, or lightheadedness. These symptoms can be an indication of dehydration, mainly low electrolytes. Since you aren't eating and losing water, you aren't getting the electrolytes your body needs to usher water into your cells. Yes, you can still be dehydrated if you drink plenty of water. To remedy those symptoms, grab a pinch or two of sea salt, place it on your tongue, and wash it down with a glass of water; it will perk you right up.

You can have a small high-fat snack under 200 calories if you need more without breaking your fast. Some examples are 1/2 of an avocado, coffee, or tea with one tbsp of heavy whipping cream, one to two tbsp of no-sugar-added nut butter, or one hard-boiled egg to help you fast a bit longer. You can use these snacks as **"training wheels"** to help you fast a bit longer. If, despite having a fasting snack, salt/electrolytes, and plenty of water, you still feel weak, tired, dizzy, have a headache or body ache, or just don't feel well, **it's time to break your fast.**

## Autophagy

Another one of the fantastic benefits of fasting is **"autophagy."** Autophagy, or **"self-eating,"** is the body's natural process of cleaning out damaged cells to regenerate newer, healthier ones, making you younger. Autophagy also plays a role in preventing diseases like cancer by causing your body to regenerate a new healthy set of stem cells and kill off the damaged ones before symptoms arise. Autophagy is a triple blessing; you get the benefits of self-healing, body fat burning, and reverse aging. Autophagy can be achieved with a **"clean fast."** Fasting only with water, unflavored mineral water, black coffee, or tea. Autophagy will kick in at about 17 hours and peak at 72 hours of fasting.

## Meal Plan to Get Started

It's time to implement what you have learned, start seeing results, and become my next success story. I am teaching you a new way of life, so take it slow and methodically. I've curated a meal plan with recipes and a grocery list to support you on your fasting and keto journey. You can access it at www.yourfatlossafter40.com. Now that you have a fasting plan, let's incorporate some fitness tips and recommendations to enhance our wellness journey.

# Chapter 8

# Fitness for Longevity

*Therefore, strengthen your feeble arms and weak knees. "Make level paths for your feet" so that the lame may not be disabled but healed. Make every effort to live in peace with everyone and to be holy; without holiness, no one will see the Lord.*

*Hebrews 12:12-14*

Welcome to the next chapter! Now that you've mastered fasting and how it pairs with a primarily keto diet and hormones, let's move into the importance of fitness on our journey together.

Researchers funded by the National Institute on Aging (NIA) have spent over four decades investigating the effects of strength training on older adults. Their findings show the importance of preserving muscle mass, improving mobility, and prolonging vibrant living. Sarcopenia, the age-related loss of muscle strength and mass, typically begins after peak muscle levels around 30 to 35 years old and accelerates after 65 for women and 70 for men.

Sarcopenia, derived from the Greek words sarx (flesh) and penia (loss), involves a decline in muscle mass, strength, and function. Although commonly associated with older adults, it can also affect middle-aged individuals. Sarcopenia leads to symptoms like weakness, fatigue, and difficulty with daily activities. It increases the risk of falls, fractures, and severe injuries and is accelerated by poor nutrition and sedentary lifestyle habits.

Embracing an active lifestyle will significantly prevent the decline of muscle strength and power associated with aging. Exercise preserves mobility, decreases the risk of falls and fractures, and promotes greater independence with aging. While aging cannot be avoided entirely, your muscle strength can be maintained through strength training exercises such as weightlifting, resistance bands, or bodyweight exercises. These activities engage muscles against resistance, triggering beneficial metabolic responses and promoting positive changes in muscle DNA.

## High-Intensity Interval Training

The workout strategy, commonly known as High-Intensity Interval Training (HIIT), stands out for its efficiency and effectiveness. Unlike traditional lengthier workouts, HIIT involves short bursts of intense exercises, like sprints or jumping jacks, followed by brief rest periods. Think of it as a workout with peaks and valleys – intense moments followed by a quick recovery. The benefit goes beyond the session; it keeps your body burning energy even after you've finished. Thanks to the afterburn effect, HIIT is a time-efficient and highly productive approach to fitness, offering a boost to your metabolism, cardiovascular, and muscular strength.

High-intensity interval training (HIIT) helps you lose fat in several ways. First, during those intense bursts of exercise, your body taps into aerobic (cardio) and anaerobic (strength) energy systems, which means it burns a lot of fuel, including stored fat. Plus, HIIT revs up your metabolism and makes your body more sensitive to insulin, which helps regulate your blood sugar levels and can lead to even more fat loss over time. Think of HIIT as a powerful tool in your fat loss arsenal. It's not just about what you burn during the workout, but also the extra fat you continue to torch even after it.

## Health Benefits of Exercising in a Fasted State

When I first heard about exercising while fasting, I thought it was crazy. Exercising on an empty stomach left me feeling drained, so I'd often need a piece of a banana to power through. However, after reading up on the research and hearing success stories, I tried it.

I started by working out before breaking my fast in the morning. A cup of black coffee beforehand gave me an extra boost of energy, and soon enough, I felt energized, and my hunger pangs disappeared. With more experience, I could work out comfortably even after an overnight water fast. Exercising in a fasted state has numerous benefits, including improved glucose tolerance, insulin sensitivity, and increased human growth hormone (HGH) release, which preserves muscle strength and encourages growth. Studies show a significant spike in HGH production after a 24-hour fast, with males experiencing a 2000% boost and females an increase of 1,300%. Fasted workouts can enhance testosterone levels, benefiting both men's and women's libido, muscle mass, and energy with age.

Many people find that exercising in a fasted state over time increases energy levels, more significant fat loss, improved muscle growth, and enhanced insulin sensitivity. If you are low on energy and struggling to get through your workout, consider adding a fasting-friendly electrolyte supplement like LMNT brand electrolyte powder to your water bottle. Alternatively, a pinch or two of sea salt can provide the boost you need to power through. Over time, your body will adapt and won't need extra helpers every time to get through it.

## How to Get the Most Out of Your Workouts

Let's explore some common workout mistakes women make and learn how to correct them.

1. Long bouts of cardio: There are better approaches than extensive steady-state cardio sessions for burning stubborn fat. This type of exercise can prompt you to hold onto fat, particularly in the lower body, and contribute to accelerated aging due to increased stress and inflammation. Instead, use HIIT workouts for that extra metabolic boost.
2. Avoiding resistance training: Fear of bulking up shouldn't keep you from resistance training. It's crucial for toning up, firming trouble areas, and boosting your metabolism to burn fat more efficiently.
3. Relying on **"woman-friendly"** workouts: Instead of opting for **"easier"** versions, focus on routines

designed to work with your body's metabolism, such as strength training and HIIT, to burn fat effectively.

4. Repeating the same workouts: Your body quickly adapts to routine, leading to plateaus in progress. Switching up your workouts every six to eight weeks is essential to continued changes.

5. Doing long workouts: More time spent exercising doesn't mean faster results. Quality over quantity is key; specific exercises can trigger a potent fat-burning effect even after your workout.

Remember, the goal is to find a balanced and effective workout routine that suits your body, is sustainable fun, and helps you achieve your fitness goals.

## Getting Started

Fitness Tips:

- Schedule your workouts into your day, and make an appointment with yourself to make them part of your routine.

- Get it done first thing in the morning before you talk yourself out of it.

- Change up your workout routine every six to eight weeks. Doing this will help you avoid hitting a plateau and boredom.

- Establish a morning routine: Establishing a morning routine can help create a consistent habit of fasted workouts.

- Celebrate small victories: Celebrate small victories to stay motivated and committed.
- Stay committed to your fitness vision for long-term success.
- Minimize insulin spikes by opting for fasted workouts in the morning.
- Exercise according to your menstrual cycle or menopausal hormone lunar cycle. The concept of "cycle syncing"—planning your workout type and intensity around your menstrual phase—has become a hot topic in the fitness world.
  - Days 1-2: Take it easy, do yoga, walk, stretch or day off.
  - Days 3-10: HIIT or intense workouts
  - Days 11-15: Heavy weights
  - Days 16-19: HIIT training
  - Days 20-30: Low intensity: Yoga, walks, light weights, Pilates, barre, leisurely bike rides

*Remember, day one is the first day you bleed.

*If you are menopausal or post-menopausal, track your cycle according to the moon/lunar phases. The new moon is your day one and two; the waxing moon is days 3-15; a full moon is days 16-19; and the waning moon is days 20-30.

You can find a sample workout calendar here to get started at www.yourfatlossafter40.com.

Now that you have learned to track and sync your cycle with your hormones, we will explore the importance of hydration and supplement recommendations for a fasting lifestyle to balance hormones and overall well-being.

Chapter 9

# Hydration and Fasting Supplementation

*After all, no one ever hated their own body, but they feed and care for*

*their body, just as Christ does the church.*

*Ephesians 5:29*

Transitioning from mindful and intuitive eating, let's discuss the importance of water and hydration, especially during fasting, and the essential supplements required for optimizing the benefits of a fasting and keto lifestyle.

Dehydration triggers hunger and sugar cravings. When people refer to initial weight loss on a low-carb diet as **'water weight,'** they're partly correct, it's a combination of stored carbohydrates and water leaving your cells. Shedding these initial pounds signifies a positive transformation as your body shifts from sugar consumption and dehydration to stable blood glucose levels and well-hydrated cells.

Staying hydrated is crucial during fasting. Aim to drink at least 64-85 ounces, or half your body weight in ounces, of water daily, especially during detox. This hydration level will help keep you satiated and contribute to a feeling of fullness. If water becomes tedious, try unsweetened electrolyte drinks for a soothing effect or a pinch of sea salt or two with your water to counteract dehydration.

Embarking on a 24- to 48-hour water fast can reset your relationship with sugar. If you feel hungry or experience low blood sugar during fasting, it's often due to insulin conditioned to metabolize carbs, dehydration, or electrolyte deficiencies. Keeping sea salt and water nearby can stabilize those energy drops. Contrary to expectations, fasting can reduce hunger and blood sugar dips. Your body has sufficient stored carbs and body fat for energy to sustain you when you are hungry.

While occasional urges to eat may arise during fasting, they're often linked to learned behaviors rather than genuine hunger. Fasting can help you recognize behavioral triggers for eating, distinguishing between physical hunger and conditioned responses driven by anxiety, depression, stress, or habit. Your stomach may growl, but you don't need food right away.

About a year ago, I decided to do my first 24-hour fast. As the evening approached, I started feeling lightheaded. Seeking advice from experienced fasters in my Facebook community, I learned that dehydration and a lack of electrolytes, particularly salt, might be the issue. Following their guidance, I took a pinch of sea salt with water and felt immediate relief. Since then, replenishing electrolytes with salt and water has become my regular practice.

## Hydration While Fasting Tips:

1. Carry a reusable water bottle with you throughout the day.

2. Enhance the taste of water by adding a slice of cucumber and mint leaves.
3. Drink water before, during, and after workouts to stay hydrated.
4. When hunger strikes, drink water first, as thirst is often mistaken for hunger.
5. Establish a drinking schedule to remind yourself to stay hydrated.
6. Opt for water when dining out to stay hydrated at no extra cost.

## Things to Consider

Whether feasting or fasting, stay ahead of dehydration by consistently drinking ample water. You lose carbohydrates and water when fasting, so staying hydrated is crucial. Since you're not getting food with electrolytes, you'll need to find other ways to maintain proper hydration.

Older adults are susceptible to dehydration symptoms due to age-related changes. Water makes up over half of your body weight and is lost daily through various means, so replenishing it is essential, particularly during hot weather, physical activity, or illness.

Proper hydration is also critical, whether you're a dedicated athlete or exercise for leisure. Drink water before, during, and after exercise to regulate body temperature, lubricate joints, transport nutrients, and support overall health. Monitor urine color as a hydration indicator—colorless or light-yellow urine signifies adequate hydration, while dark yellow or amber may indicate dehydration.

Dehydration occurs when the fluid loss exceeds intake, affecting body function. Symptoms include:

- Dizziness or lightheaded feeling
- Nausea or vomiting
- Headache
- Dry lips
- Muscle cramps and weakness
- Dry mouth
- Joint ache
- Lack of sweating
- A fast heartbeat
- Severe dehydration (mental confusion, weakness, and loss of consciousness, requiring immediate medical attention)

Meeting your daily hydration requirements can be manageable with these five tips:

1. **Carry a Water Bottle**: Sip a cute reusable water bottle throughout the day.
2. **Set Reminders**: Use phone alarms or apps to remind you to drink water regularly. Example (drink 32oz between 7 am and 12 pm, 12 pm and 4 pm, and 4-8 pm). Don't worry; your body will adapt within seven days, and you won't have to run to the bathroom as often.

3. **Eat Water-Rich Foods:** Add a packet of LMT to add flavor and interest.

4. **Make it Fun:** Customize your water bottle and consider adding cute accents and decorations. Add slices of cucumber and ice to keep it cool and refreshing, making drinking water more enjoyable.

5. **Hydrate Before Meals**: Have a glass of water before each meal to ensure regular intake.

## Fasting Support Supplements

Here is a list of the supplements I recommend to help you optimize your fasting experience. Links to products can be found at www.yourfatlossafter40.com

- MCT oil: MCT (Medium-Chain Triglycerides) oil is a concentrated source of fats that are easily converted into energy during fasting. It supports fat metabolism, boosts quick energy, and enhances brain clarity.

- LMNT minerals: LMNT minerals, including sodium, potassium, and magnesium, are crucial for electrolyte balance. They help prevent dehydration and muscle cramps commonly associated with fasting.

- Vitamin B: Vitamin B plays a vital role in energy metabolism. Supplements can help maintain energy levels and emotional stability while fasting and support overall well-being when nutrient intake is limited.

- Magnesium Glycinate: Magnesium is an essential mineral that supports various bodily functions, including muscle and nerve functions. It can help alleviate muscle cramps, decrease sugar cravings, help with sleep, and support relaxation during fasting.

- Glucose Monitor or Ketone Monitor: Using a ketone and blood sugar monitor gives valuable insights into how your body responds to the transition into ketosis and the effects of different foods on your blood sugar levels. It helps me understand what breaks a fast and which foods support ketosis. As a quick rule of thumb, a 10mg/dl increase in blood sugar indicates a broken fast. These supplements can enhance your fasting experience by providing essential nutrients, supporting energy levels, and ensuring a well-balanced electrolyte status.

Now that you know why you need to get your body moving and what to take to optimize fasting, prepare to learn to listen and be mindful of what your body tells you in the next chapter.

# Chapter 10

# Mindful and Intuitive Eating

*The Lord is my shepherd, I lack nothing. He makes me lie down in green pastures, he leads me beside quiet waters, he refreshes my soul. He guides me along the right path for his name's sake. Even though I walk through the darkest valley, I will fear no evil, for you are with me; your rod and your staff, they comfort me.*

*Psalm 23:1-4*

Following fitness comes mindful and intuitive eating. Mindfully staying in tune with your body's requests regarding food and fitness is also essential to longevity.

Let's start with the difference between a traditional diet and a lifestyle approach—the basis lies in your relationship with food and your flexibility. Are you open to going rogue if your body says, *"I need an extra piece of fruit,"* even when it's not part of the meal plan or when you've already exhausted the carbs available for the day on your keto meal plan?

This program was never intended to be a quick-fix weight loss solution with rigid rules. Instead, it is designed to tap into the infinite wisdom God created in our bodies to serve our ultimate level of wellness best. There may be days when you must rely on your body's wisdom and test its limits according to your physical symptoms.

On some days, fasting may feel like a total breeze; on others, it might be more challenging to reach your 16-hour mark. Some days, a keto diet feels fantastic, while on other days, you may crave an extra serving or two of veggies or that apple you've been eyeing on your countertop. That is all completely okay and welcome.

Remember that your dietary habits should make you feel better, not worse. If you are fasting and feel bad, break your fast and enjoy a deliciously nourishing whole-food meal. After all, your body may need extra fruit or veggies to restore certain hormones. The same goes for exercise. Push yourself to boost your fitness and strengthen your body, but listen to your body if you don't feel well or are in pain. Take it easy, stop, and return to it the next day, or seek medical attention to address any imbalances in your anatomy.

## Listening to Your Body

I was introduced to mindful and intuitive eating more than twenty years ago while I was in the eating disorders treatment program. It was a new concept back then, but it has become a mainstream movement for those who want to break free from dieting. Mindful and intuitive eating helps you to get back into the in-between. At that time, mindful eating was my door to liberation from restrictive dieting. I discovered that food didn't always have to dictate my weight or put me at risk of gaining weight. I allowed myself to eat according to what felt best for me without feeling guilty or fearing the consequences.

Since starting my career as a dietitian 27 years ago, I've embraced teaching mindful and intuitive eating to my clients and groups. Unlike conventional diets that dictate strict food rules, mindful and intuitive eating focuses on how food makes you feel. It prioritizes listening to your body's signals, such as feeling energized after a balanced meal rather than sluggish after a carb-heavy one.

## Mindful Eating

We live in a society where extremes in food and body weight prevail: either very underweight or very overweight, with patterns of relentless restrictive eating or excessive overeating. Let's start with mindful eating; it involves being mentally and physically present, allowing you to truly experience your food's taste, texture, aroma, and colors. Mindful eating includes a healthy weight management approach, breaking up with the scale if you are in a toxic relationship with it, reducing stress, connecting with your body's real needs, appreciating food more, disrupting emotional eating habits, increasing motivation to exercise, and interrupting mindless relationships with food.

Mindful eating is about:

- Eating slowly and without distraction.
- Listening to physical hunger cues and eating until you're full.

- Distinguishing between true hunger and non-hunger triggers for eating.
- Engaging your senses by noticing colors, smells, sounds, textures, and flavors.
- Learning to cope with guilt and anxiety about food.
- Eating to maintain overall health and well-being.
- Noticing the effects food has on your feelings and figure.
- Appreciate your food and those who grew it.

Practicing mindful eating involves being aware of your food choices and eating experience, reconnecting with your body's cues for hunger and satiety, and moving away from fixation on numbers and measurements.

To practice mindful eating, let's go through a quick exercise together. This step-by-step exercise will only take a few minutes.

1. Prepare for the exercise: Find a small piece of food, like a raisin, a nut, or a small piece of a cookie. Select something you enjoy, as mindful eating is not about deprivation.
2. Engage your senses: Look at the food. Notice its texture and color. Close your eyes and explore it with your sense of touch, noting hardness, softness, graininess, or stickiness. Use one sense at a time, practicing without judgment.
3. Smell the food: Use your sense of smell to explore the food's aroma before eating.

4. Begin eating: Regardless of size, take at least two bites to finish your chosen food. Chew slowly and attentively, savoring the sensory experience of tasting and chewing.

5. Focus on texture: Pay attention to the texture in your mouth. Slowly finish the first bite for about 20 seconds, fully aware of the sensations.

6. Take the second bite: Similar to the first, chew the second and last bite slowly, fully aware of sensations, flavor changes, and swallowing. Notice the sensations and movements of chewing, the changing flavor, and the act of swallowing. Pay attention, moment by moment.

Embracing mindfulness in your diet goes beyond eating slowly; it involves a thoughtful approach to thoughts, emotions, and bodily sensations related to eating. This practice can help overcome cravings and stress-induced eating. While eating this slowly isn't always necessary, starting with a deliberate pace can enhance mindfulness.

## Intuitive Eating

As a broader concept, intuitive eating encourages tuning into your body's cues, embracing momentary cravings, and choosing what intuitively feels right. It involves selecting foods you genuinely desire, experiencing them fully without distractions, and appreciating the fullness they bring. Let go of judgment and savor the taste. It means listening to your body and choosing foods that make you feel your best—foods that bring enjoyment and pleasure and promote healthy weight and good health.

## Mindful and Intuitive Eating Practice

For today's assignment, practice mindful and intuitive eating during your meals. Enjoy one breakfast, lunch, dinner, and snack mindfully, choosing foods that make you feel your best. Repeat this exercise at least four times, sitting down without distractions and journaling your hunger levels before and after each meal. It's a great way to integrate mindful and intuitive eating into your daily routine. Get ready to take the next step as we dive into advanced fasting techniques in the upcoming chapter.

## Chapter 11

# My Top Four Tips for Maximizing Fasting Results

*May he give you the desire of your heart*

*and make all your plans succeed.*

*Psalm 20:4*

Now that you've learned the importance of incorporating mindful and intuitive eating let's explore strategies to enhance your fasting journey further.

As you learned in Chapter 7, fasting can be a powerful tool for improving health, boosting energy, and promoting weight loss. Still, it can also present challenges, especially when you want to maximize your results. Incorporating advanced strategies into your fasting routine can boost your body's ability to adapt, overcome common setbacks, and achieve your goals more efficiently. In this chapter, I'm excited to share my top four tips for optimizing your fasting experience and unlocking its full potential. Let's go.

## Tip #1: Understanding Appetite Hormones

When your body is accustomed to burning carbohydrates for fuel, even short periods without food can trigger hunger, driven by the hormone ghrelin. Based on your regular eating schedule, the hormone ghrelin is released, causing hunger pangs in waves every three to four hours. However, as you adapt to fasting, these ghrelin waves become less frequent and eventually stop once you enter ketosis. Quality sleep also lowers ghrelin secretion and reduces late-night hunger pangs.

Leptin, another appetite hormone produced by fat cells, signals your brain to stop eating and is triggered by fats and proteins but not carbs. Eating healthy fats and proteins can improve satiety, but stress and excessive carbohydrate intake can lead to leptin resistance, causing you to eat more often. Combining fasting with a diet high in fat (60%), moderate in protein (30%), and low in carbs (10%) enhances your body's satiety signals, allowing you to go longer without food.

Next, insulin regulates blood sugar levels and helps cells absorb carbs for energy. Excess insulin stimulation from carbohydrate foods and excess protein over 30 grams per meal signals your body to store energy as body fat. While fasting, your body depletes its stored carbohydrate reserves and burns fat for fuel. Insulin resistance (pre-diabetes) is an imbalance of this digestive hormone. It is common in women over 40 to have ineffective or depleted insulin levels, but it can be improved with regular fasting. By depleting carb stores, you can increase insulin sensitivity, lower blood sugar levels, and promote body fat loss, reducing the risk of type 2 diabetes and cardiovascular issues.

Spacing out your meals with daily fasting (12-24 hours) is excellent for curbing impulsive eating. You are giving your stomach's vagus nerve a break. The vagus nerve signals hunger and satiety between your brain and gut, significantly influencing your eating behavior.

## Tip #2: How to Overcome Persistent Morning Hunger

I struggled with persistent morning gnawing hunger in the first five months of my fasting journey. I thought this was normal, and when I asked my husband and the fasting group, they said they had not experienced that sensation. I did some research and realized my symptoms could be a gut health issue caused by an overgrowth of harmful bacteria. To address this, I adjusted my fasting routine by breaking my fasts with gut-friendly foods like sauerkraut or kimchi, along with avocado or a cup of plain kefir. I also made sure to close my eating window by 7 pm to avoid acid buildup caused by food in my stomach while I slept. Within a few days, the annoying morning hunger disappeared. This experience taught me the importance of nurturing gut health to eliminate excess hunger.

## Tip #3: Recommendations for Improving Your Fasting Experience

**Gradually Extend Fasting Windows**: Start with a 12-hour fasting window and progressively increase it to 14 hours with a 10-hour eating window, then to 16/8, 18/6, and 20/4 intervals. Try extended periods like 23/1, 36-hour, or 48-hour fasts. For a more advanced approach, experiment with a three-day water fast a few times a year—alternate fasting patterns to add flexibility.

**Stay Hydrated**: Drink water regularly, especially while fasting and before, during, and after workouts. When hunger strikes, drink water first to distinguish between thirst and hunger. If energy levels drop, consider electrolyte supplements like magnesium, LMNT, or a pinch of sea salt.

**Shake Up Your Fasting Routine:** Experiment with different fasting schedules if fat loss slows. Try taking a five-day fasting break or incorporating a 36-hour fast during the first ten days of your cycle or when estrogen is high. This approach can help reset metabolic pathways and promote more efficient fat release.

**Start with Shorter Fasts:** If hunger is challenging, start with a shorter 12-14-hour fast while maintaining a hormone-building keto diet. Once comfortable, gradually extend fasts to 18-24 hours once a week, using a fasting snack if needed. You know you've entered ketosis when hunger diminishes, your brain is clear, and your energy is high.

**Prioritize Quality Nutrition:** During your eating window, incorporate probiotics and prebiotic foods to support gut health, and consider a parasite/candida cleanse to eliminate harmful organisms. These practices can alleviate hunger and promote overall wellness.

## Tip #4: Easily Enter Ketosis

Keeping blood sugar levels low and preventing insulin spikes is critical to accessing and burning body fat. When insulin levels rise, your body switches from burning fat to using carbohydrates for energy. Here are some strategies to deplete stored carbohydrates and quickly transition into fat-burning mode:

- **Limit Carbohydrate Intake**: To deplete glycogen stores, reduce your carb intake to 10% of your diet. Opt for low-carb foods like vegetables, nuts, seeds, and healthy fats.

- **Engage in Exercise:** Physical activity, especially high-intensity (HIIT) workouts, 3-5 days/week, can quickly deplete glycogen stores in your muscles, promoting fat burning.

- **Intermittent Fasting:** Fasting periods help lower insulin levels and deplete glycogen stores, facilitating the transition into ketosis.

- **Stay Hydrated**: Drinking plenty of water supports glycogen breakdown and elimination through urine.

- **Prioritize Sleep**: Quality sleep is essential for regulating insulin levels and promoting fat metabolism. Aim for seven to nine hours of uninterrupted sleep each night.

- **Infrared Sauna**: Infrared sauna sessions enhance the release of stored fats, supporting detoxification and weight loss efforts.

- **Sun Exposure:** Spending 15-20 min in the sun, particularly during summer, breaks down fat cells under the skin, leading to more significant body fat loss.

- **Dry Brushing:** Practice dry brushing before showering. Using a round bristle brush, gently brush your skin from your outer limbs toward your heart to promote lymphatic drainage and help break down fats and toxins stored in the skin.

Combine these techniques to significantly boost your overall metabolic health and overcome stubborn fat loss plateaus. As always, listen to your body and learn from it. Never ignore pain or discomfort that is beyond your normal level. Our objective is to strengthen our bodies, not weaken them. These additional strategies are your key to a successful fasting journey. Let's make the most of this transformative experience together. In this next chapter, I will share how to put everything you have learned together to become the fit, fabulous, and fierce woman over 40 you desire to be.

## Chapter 12

# Fit, Fabulous, and Fierce Over 40

*For you created my inmost being;*

*you knit me together in my mother's womb.*

*I praise you because I am fearfully and wonderfully made;*

*your works are wonderful, I know that full well.*

*Psalm 139:13-14*

Congratulations on reaching the culmination of this journey, soaking in the invaluable lessons that have both challenged and transformed you. These experiences have moved you toward becoming the fit, fabulous, and ageless beauty you aspire to be.

On our journey together, you have learned the importance of:

- Rewiring your thoughts and mindset for success.
- Casting your vision.
- Annual spring cleaning for your body. Including a liver detox and candida/parasite cleanse.
- Fasting with your hormone cycle and keto-style eating with the addition of hormone-boosting foods.
- Fitness routine for longevity

- Hydration and supplements to support fasting and your health.
- Mindful and intuitive eating (listening to your body).
- Strategies for maximizing fasting benefits for body fat loss
- Living in grace

In this program, I have also taught you to embrace the importance of rejecting all-or-nothing thinking, focusing instead on love and self-care, not fear or condemnation. Life is a journey of constant evolution, with our bodies adapting to changing needs and desires. Falling off track and getting back on isn't failure but resilience—an opportunity for growth. Each day offers a fresh start, a chance to nourish our bodies as a form of reverence for the divine temple they are, leading to both feeling and looking our best.

Unlike diets, which often induce stress and emotional turmoil, grace embodies love, connection, and understanding. It feels effortless, peaceful, and free from judgment. With grace, we transition from habits that no longer serve us to those that do. As strong, compassionate women, we rise above diet culture, prioritizing genuine wellness and well-being.

Following practical steps is excellent for weight loss, but true transformation begins with your self-talk. To begin to accept God's grace on your journey, start by identifying the lies— those thoughts misaligned with God's Word. When you hear a whisper telling you that you're not good enough or can't go on vacation until you lose weight, recognize that it's not the voice of God. Pay attention, and you'll notice a common theme: the overriding voice is one of shame.

While living out a fasting lifestyle, your weight will ebb and flow. You are in this for the long haul, and over time, despite the ebbs and flows, you will see a gradual decline. Plus, you can adjust your eating times and use some of my tips to make subtle changes to your lifestyle habits that will get you back on track with your weight loss.

## Bringing it All Together: Top Ten Lifestyle Tips

Before we finish, I want to conclude with my top ten wellness lifestyle tips. These tips are all about how to become the fit, fabulous, and fierce woman this program promised you to be.

**Tip 1: Embrace circadian rhythm fasting by aligning your eating patterns with the sun.** When the sun shines, melatonin (the sleep hormone) is low, and insulin operates optimally. As the sun sets, melatonin rises, and insulin resistance increases, leading to heightened fat storage—especially with the consumption of carbs, alcohol, and protein during the evening hours.

**Tip 2: Sync Fasting with Lunar Phases.**

Align your fasting routine with the moon's phases, recognizing its impact on hormonal cycles. Excessive blue light exposure, especially from screens, disrupts your natural connection to the moon and sun. Wear blue light glasses when looking at a screen when it is dark outside or if you need more sunlight exposure.

If you're unfamiliar with your hormonal cycles or lack a regular one, use the moon's phases as a fasting guide.

Align your fasting strategy with the phases of your menstrual cycle:

- **Days 1-10:** High energy, mental clarity. Opt for fat-burning exercises and extended fasts with elevated estrogen and lower progesterone.
- **Days 11-15:** Boost creativity and energy. Engage in more intense workouts to capitalize on enhanced endurance. Keep fasting for no more than 15 hours.
- **Days 16-19:** Return to your high-energy workout and tap into extended fasting.
- **Days 20-first day of the period:** Elevated progesterone. Experience lower energy and a preference for carbs. Take a break from fasting (no more than 13 hours), include healthy fats, and supplement with magnesium for hormonal balance during this phase and low-intensity exercise like walking, yoga, or stretching.

**Tip 3: Change Up Your Fasting and Clear Toxins to Break Through Plateaus.**

Try a 36-hour fast followed by a 12-hour fast. Check armpits and above-collarbones for pockets or pits containing trapped toxins. Remember, the more body fat you have, the more estrogen-dominant you may be. Incorporate practices like sweating and dry brushing and limit alcohol and processed foods to prevent the re-accumulation of lost fat.

**Tip 4: Autophagy Fast vs. Ketosis Fast.** Yoshinori Ohsumi won a Nobel Prize for uncovering autophagy – your body's cleanup crew. Increase autophagy using High-Intensity Interval Training (HIIT) and add foods that increase autophagy to get the most benefit. It's like treating your cells to a spa day, working wonders to reverse aging and ease inflammation. Ketosis is flipping a switch to burn fat instead of carbs. Say goodbye to carb burning and insulin resistance, and help to your journey to becoming a fat burner.

**Tip 5: Change Your Workouts Every Six Weeks and Sync them with your Hormonal Cycle.**

Keeping your workouts fresh and exciting is key to sustained progress. Incorporate a mix of High-Intensity Interval Training (HIIT) to boost your metabolism and strength exercises to build muscle and boost metabolic flexibility. Remember to add some fun activities to keep things enjoyable. Switching up your routine every six weeks prevents plateaus, challenges your body, and ensures you stay engaged on your fitness journey. Training smart around your menstrual cycle can help you feel more empowered in your wellness journey, optimize your workouts, and enhance your longevity.

**Tip 6: Live Out the Vision for Yourself.**

When faced with challenges or temptations, remember your "why," your vision for yourself. Enjoying a fasting snack is okay; the key is mindful choices. Bring God into the process and count on Him for breakthroughs. Your journey is not just about a physical transformation but also about lining up with your deeper purpose. Stay focused on the vision and let it guide you through your new fasting lifestyle.

## Tip 7: Live by the 80/20 Rule.

Keep 80% of your food choices on plan while allowing 20% flexibility. Eating this way will give you a healthy balance between structure and adaptability. Fully embrace the freedom to indulge occasionally, understanding that consistency matters more than occasional pleasure foods in the long run.

## Tip 8: Know When to Stop Fasting.

Pay attention to your body's signals and stop fasting if you experience low urine output, dizziness, stomach pain, racing heart rate, extreme hunger, nausea, insomnia, or unresolved weakness, even with additional water and electrolytes (sodium, magnesium, and potassium).

Avoid fasting if you're experiencing missed periods, exaggerated PMS, pregnancy, breastfeeding, psychologically detrimental disturbances, your doctor says you need to, or hormonal imbalances.

There's no shame in breaking a fast early — it's not a competition. Fasting takes practice, and you can try again when you feel ready. The goal is to improve your health, not hinder it.

## Tip 9: Embrace Your Authentic Self and Stay in Your Lane

I'm saving the best and most important for last. First, use your scale only if it helps and does not hinder your mental and physical progress (which is rare). Otherwise, I invite you to throw it out the window, toss it in the trash, or smash it into small pieces (with shoes, gloves, and goggles on). This program is a new lifestyle, and your weight will fluctuate, especially during maintenance.

In this last step, let's look into your heart. You, my friend, are a masterpiece seen through God's eyes. Your unique and radiant spirit is the essence of your beauty. Living authentically means running your race, staying in your lane, and being your best version, not copying someone else. Embrace every aspect of your beauty, inside and out, knowing your identity in Christ. Your journey is about discovering and celebrating the incredible person you are.

## Cheryl's Journey to Renewal and Balance

Over two years ago, I met Cheryl at my church's annual women's retreat. She eagerly joined my 21-Day Sugar Detox Group, where she reversed pre-diabetic symptoms and chronic high blood sugar. Inspired by her recent success, she embarked on my journey on November 6, 2022, starting at 198.1 pounds. By the end of the detox, she lost 15 pounds and broke her sugar addiction, feeling incredible.

However, after a challenging winter with cabin fever and late-night snacking, her weight began to climb again. Determined not to regress, she joined my Ageless Body Blueprint program. As of May 10th, she reached 178 pounds, halfway to her goal of losing 20 pounds. Intermittent fasting has been pivotal, helping her cut out late-night snacks and reshape her mindset.

This holistic approach silenced negative self-talk and taught her to appreciate her body at every stage. She's incorporated prayer, internal growth, and balanced hormone management through diet and supplements like magnesium.

At 58, she said, *"I feel as vibrant as in my 20s. Beyond weight loss, the real triumph lies in achieving a life balance and reshaping my relationship with food."* Cheryl's journey shows that taking that first step and staying committed can lead to the transformative results that you desire.

Now, it is time to create your testimonial of triumph!

When you put the book down, join my community for added accountability and support to keep flaming your fire. Join my **"Over 40 and Fabulous"** Facebook group at https://www.facebook.com/groups/fatlossover40solution. I also encourage you to join my online course group for this book. We are a tight community of women going through this journey together. You can join our weekly Q&A calls to connect with fellow group members and me, share your progress, and uplift others on similar journeys. Together, let's continue toward holistic well-being. Visit my YouTube channel https://www.youtube.com/@CynthiaARay for guidance, and expect new content in the group or my online course.

If everything you've learned here has stirred a desire in you to deepen your connection with God or start a relationship with Jesus, I invite you to pray this prayer:

*"Lord, I'm sorry for how I've treated myself and my past actions. I need a savior to help me break free from the struggles in my mind. I long for the freedom and peace Cynthia described in this book. Please come into my heart and lead my life. Thank you for sacrificing your life on the cross and defeating death over 2,000 years ago so that I can live in peace and eternity with you, free from fear of death. I want to become the person you've designed me to be. Thank you, Jesus. Amen."*

If you've prayed this prayer, reach out to a friend or me to celebrate with you. We'll support you and help you grow closer to God, experiencing all the blessings He has in store. ♥ It's time to get out there and change your life!

# Additional Resources

# The Fasting Cycle

| Day 1-10 - Period starts on Day 1 | | Day 11-15 | Day 16-19 | Day 20-30 |
|---|---|---|---|---|
| **POWER PHASE** | | **MANIFESTATION (OVULATION)** | **POWER PHASE 2** | **NURTURE PHASE** |
| Intermittent Fasting 13-72 hours | | Intermittent Fasting 13-15 hours max | Intermittent Fasting 13-72 hours | NO FASTING |
| **Feed: Keto** | | **Feed: Hormone Feasting** | **Feed: Keto** | **Feed: Hormone Feast** |
| Insulin and Estrogen<br>**Keto**<br>50 gr net carbs<br>75 gr protein<br>>60% from good fat<br><br>**Good Fats**<br>Olive Oil<br>Flaxseed oil<br>Sesame oil<br>Avocado | **Seeds and nuts**<br>Almonds, Cashews; Roasted peanuts, Pine nuts, Pumpkin seeds, Sunflower seeds, Walnuts, Sesame seeds<br><br>**Legumes**<br>Peas, Chickpeas, Soybeans, Kidney Beans, Lentils, Pinto beans, edamame, Tofu<br><br>**Fruits and vegs**<br>cabbage, Onion, Garlic, Zucchini Broccoli, Cauliflower, Strawberries, Blueberries, Cranberries | Estrogen & Testost<br>**Hormone Feasting**<br>**100-150 gr net carbs**<br>**50 gr protein**<br>**Heathy fates**<br><br>Pumpkin seeds<br>Navy beans<br>Organic Tofu<br><br>**Three P's**<br>Probiotic<br>Polyphenol<br>Prebiotic<br><br>**Root veg & Fruit** | **Good Fats**<br>Olive oil, Flaxseed oil, Sesame Oil, Avocado<br><br>**Seeds and nuts**<br>Almonds, Cashews, Roasted peanuts, Pine nuts, Pumpkin seeds, Sunflower seeds, Walnuts, Sesame seeds<br><br>**Legumes**<br>Peas, Chickpeas, Soybeans, Kidney beans, Lentils, Pinto beans, Edamame, Tofu<br><br>**Fruits and vegs**<br>Cabbage, Onion, Garlic, Zucchini, Broccoli, Cauliflower, Strawberries, Blueberries, Cranberries | **Root Vegetables**<br>White potatoes, Red potatoes, Yams, Beets, Turnips, Fennel, Pumpkin, Butternut, Squash, Acorn Squash<br><br>**Cruciferous Vegetables**<br>Brussel sprouts, Cauliflower, Broccoli<br><br>**Tropical fruits**<br>Bananas, Mangoes, Papaya<br><br>**Citrus Fruits**<br>Orange, Grapefruit, Lemon, Lime<br><br>**Seeds**<br>Sunflower, Flax, Sesame<br><br>**Legumes**<br>Chickpea, Kidney beans, Black Beans |
| *ALL MONTH: Quinoa, Mushrooms, Chia, Tofu, Olive oil, Avocado oil, Coconut oil, Sesame oil, Avocados, Olives, Coconut, Raw nut butters, Three P's | | | | |
| D1-2: No exercise or Low intensity | **HIIT TRAINING Tabata** | Heavy Weights | **HIIT TRAINING Tabata** | Low Intensity: Yoga, walks, hikes, barre, Pilates, lighter weights |

# Foods That Support Hormones

| Keto Food | Hormone feasting food | ESTROGEN foods | PROGESTERONE Foods | The three P's (All month Long) | Food to avoid |
|---|---|---|---|---|---|
| Power Phase (Day 1-10 & Day 16-19) | Manifestation Phase (Day 11-15) & Nurture | **Good Fats** Olive oil, Flaxseed oil, Sesame oil, Avocados | **Root Vegetables** White potatoes, Red potatoes, Sweet potatoes, Yams, Beets, Turnips, Fennel, Pumpkin, Butternut Squash, Acorn Squash | **PROBIOTIC** Sauerkraut, Kimchi, Pickles, Yogurt, Kombucha, Kefir dairy, Kefir water | **Food to avoid** Partially hydrogenated oils Corn oil Cottonseed oil Vegetable oil Soybean oil Safflower oil Sunflower oil, Bread, Pasta, Crackers, Desserts, Gluten free flours Honey (reset) Coconut sugar (reset) Artificial Colors and Flavors Red or Blue Dyes Saccharin NutraSweet Splenda Refined Flours and oils Alcohol |
| Fasts 13-72 hours | Fast +15 hours | **Seeds and Nuts** Brazil nuts, Almonds, Cashews, Roasted Cashews, Pine nuts, Pumpkin seeds, Sunflower seeds, Walnuts, Sesame Seeds | **Cruciferous Vegs** Brussel Sprouts, Cauliflower, Broccoli | **PREBIOTIC** Onions, Jerusalem artichokes, Garlic, Leeks, Asparagus, Tomatoes, Leafy greens, Red Kidney beans, Chia, Chickpeas, Lentils, Split peas, Cashews, Pistachios, hummus, Berries, Apples, Cherries, Mango, Kiwi, Pears, Hemp & Flax seeds,, Chicory root, Dandelion root, Konjac root, Burdock root | |
| **Hormones: Insulin and estrogen** | **Hormones: Estrogen & Testosterone (MP) Cortisol & Progesterone (Nurture)** | **Legumes** Peas, Chickpeas, Soybeans, Kidney beans, Lentils, Pinto beans, Edamame, Tofu | **Tropical fruits** Bananas, Mangos, Papaya | | |
| **Food plan:** 50 gr net carbs 75 gr protein > 60% from good fat | **Food plan:** 100-150 gr net carbohydrates 50 gr protein Healthy fats as desired | **Fruits and vegs** Cabbage, Onion, Garlic, Zucchini, Broccoli, Cauliflower, Strawberries, Blueberries, Cranberries | **Citrus Fruit** Orange, Grapefruit Lemon, Lime | **POLYPHENOL** Artichoke hearts, Broccoli, Brussel sprouts, Cloves, Saffron, Oregano, Rosemary, Sage, Thyme, Basil, Cinnamon, Cumin, Curry, Dark Chocolate, Blueberries, Raw Hazelnuts & Pecans, Cauliflower, Olives, Parsley, Red wine, Shallots, Raw chestnuts | **Food to add** Good Fats: **Olive oil** **Flaxseed oil** **Pumpkin oil** **Nut Butter** **Olives** **Avocados** Grass-fed beef Bison Turkey Chicken Pork Egg Charcuterie |
| **Seeds and nuts** Almonds, Cashews, Roasted peanuts, Pine nuts, Pumpkin seeds, Sunflower seeds, Walnuts, Sesame seeds<br>**Legumes** Peas, Chickpeas, Soybeans, Kidney beans, Lentils, Pinto beans, Edamame, Tofu<br>**Fruits and vegs** Cabbage, Onion, Garlic, Zucchini, Broccoli, Cauliflower, Strawberries, Blueberries, Cranberries | **Cruciferous vegs** Broccoli, Brussel sprouts, Cauliflower<br>**Green leafy vegs** Arugula, Friese, Kale, Watercress<br>**Seeds** Sesame seeds, Flax Seeds<br>**Fermented Foods** Sauerkraut, Kimchi, Yogurt<br>**Berries** Blueberries, Raspberries, Boysenberries<br>Apples<br>Green & Dandelion teas<br>Salmon<br>**Spices** Turmeric, Cumin, Saffron, Dill | | **Seeds** Sunflower, Flax, Sesame<br>**Legumes** Chickpeas, Kidney beans, Black beans<br>**Good Fats** Pumpkin Oil, Sunflower oil<br>Sprouts | **All month long foods:** **Quinoa, Chia, Mushrooms, Tofu, Avocado, Olives, Raw nut butters.** | |

# How to Break a Fast

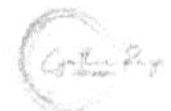

| Restore Gut | Protein | Keep Fat Burning |
|---|---|---|
| • Probiotic Rich Foods (good bacteria)<br><br>• Prebiotic (Grow microbes to boost immune system - Mood enhancing - break down estrogen)<br><br>• Polyphenol (Repairs mucusol lining - Best for low energy, chronic pain, brain fog or leaky gut)<br><br>Fermented yogurt<br>Sauerkraut<br>Kombucha<br>Seeds and oils<br><br>Bone Broth | **Muscle Building**<br>Stimulates mTOR<br>30gr Protein<br><br>Protein shake (pea, hemp)<br>Chickpea<br>Lima bean<br>Quinoa<br>Avocado<br><br>**High Protein veggies**<br>Broccoli, peas, sprouts, Brussel sprouts, mushrooms<br><br>Beef sticks<br>Beef Jerky<br>Slicked Deli Meats<br>Chicken Breasts<br>Turkey<br>Grass-fed beef | **Weight loss**<br>Fat stabilizes blook sugar the most<br><br>Avocado<br>Raw nuts<br>Nut butters<br>Olives<br><br>Bone Broth |

| Things that don't take you out of a fasted state | Fasting snack (Only if REALLY needed!) |
|---|---|
| Water<br>Black Coffee<br>Coffee with full fat milk<br>Tea<br>Oils (incl. Flaxseed oil and MCT)<br>Mineral water<br>Fresh pressed ginger and lemon drink | Nut butter - 2T<br>MCT oil - 1T<br>Seed oil - 1T<br>Grass-fed cream - 1/4 cup |

## Break Longer Fast (48+ Hours)

| Step 1 | Step 2 | Step 3 | Step 4 |
|---|---|---|---|
| **Drink a cup of ANY Broth**<br><br>WAIT AN HOUR | **Eat a PROBIOTIC rich meal with fat**<br><br>Fermented yogurt<br>Sauerkraut<br>Kombucha<br>Olives<br><br>WAIT AND HOUR | **STEAMED VEGGIES with drizzled oil**<br><br>Small sweet potato<br>Purple sweet potato with grass-fed butter<br><br>WAIT AN HOUR | **Eat 30gr of protein to build muscle!**<br><br>Regular size meal now Ok!<br><br>HEALING TAKES TIME! |

# Acknowledgments

To my Father God for giving me the desire to inspire and educate others from my overflowing passion. His love, support, and reminders in the middle of the night and early mornings of who I am and what my mission is kept me going. For inspiring me to share the beautiful intricacies He created in our bodies with the world. The delicate balance between health, wellness, and self-love and care. Thank you for guiding me when I lost my way and bringing so many beautiful people to support, encourage, and educate me beyond the education I could get at any university.

To my loving and supportive husband, Corey. He is patient with me, doing his best to keep up with my ever-changing, passionate ideas.

He was as essential to completing this book as I was. Thank you, Corey, for doing errands, taking the kids out, and doing the dishes so I could write and edit. Your loving support means everything.

To my children, Cooper, Camble, and Charlotte, for keeping me on my toes and remaining patient when I wasn't available or my brain was too tired. I am thankful to be your teacher, and you keeping me excited about learning and teaching.

To Donna Partow, thank you for responding to God's calling and making yourself available to share your book-writing and publishing wisdom. I love that you challenge and inspire me to think bigger, beyond the books. Thank you for believing in me and my message for the world. I am grateful for your encouragement and deadlines to continue on the path of excellence as the only option.

To my lovely, talented, and super intelligent friends Cyndi Rai, Christine Liepins, and Karin Rudolf, for taking the time to review this book with a critical eye to make it perfect.

Lastly, I want to thank all the amazing women who have continued with me beyond the "21-Day Sugar Detox" and through the "Ageless Body Blueprint" course, inspiring me to give you more. Cheers to my Fit, Fabulous, and FIERCE tribe of women over 40. Thank you, ladies. I am grateful to have you in my life.

# About the Author

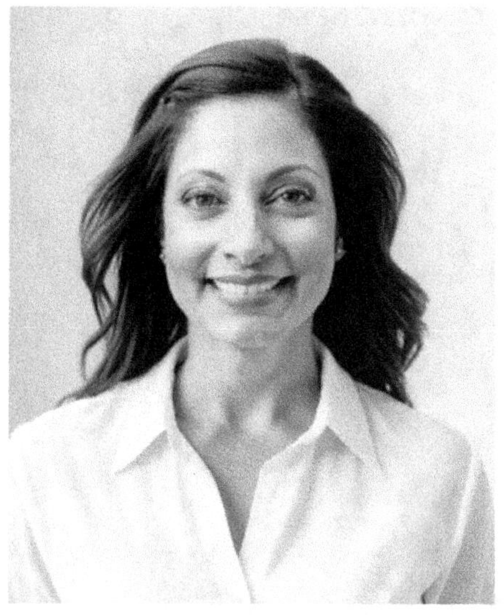

I am a homeschooling mom of three and married to my loving husband, Corey. I enjoy exercise and need it daily for my mental health. I am thankful for my family and the freedom to live where we want.

I am a registered and licensed dietitian and fitness specialist with over twenty-five years of experience treating clients in private practice, virtual programs, and courses. In addition to treating clinical conditions, I specialize in helping clients achieve their best health and enjoy a peaceful relationship with food and balanced eating.

I am passionate about learning, sharing, supporting, encouraging, and educating the community for better physical, emotional, and spiritual health.

# Other Books by Cynthia A. Ray

## *The 21-Day Sugar Detox*

### Crush Your Sugar Cravings Now!

What if you could retrain your body to crave *healthy foods* for a change? Now you can!

*The 21-Day Sugar Detox* combines the best strategies from diets that work fast for women. It combines:

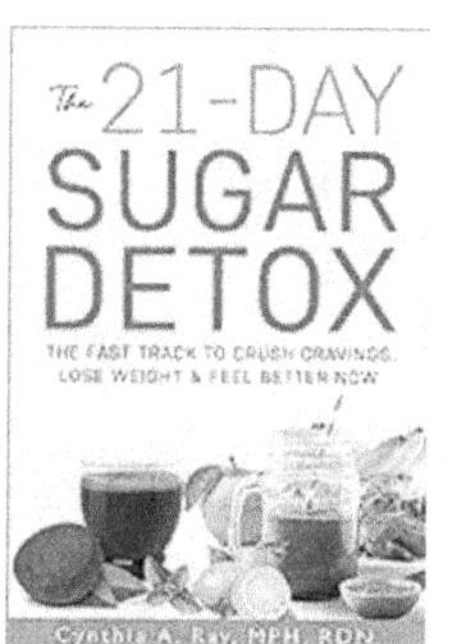


- Paleo-style eating plan
- Detox drinks & green smoothies
- Anti-inflammatory foods & effective supplements
- Delicious low-carb recipes that promote healthy weight loss

Each day includes practical ideas to break the vicious cycle that drives carb addiction. And because this book is primarily for Christian women, there's a brief devotional, prayer, and journal prompt. For the past 25 years, Cynthia Ray has been helping women heal in spirit, soul, and body. Now it's YOUR turn. Her proven approach will show you exactly how to transform your health from the inside out, starting today!

Grab your copy here: www.21dayswithoutsugar.com

# Pay It Forward

Thank you from the bottom of my heart for reading my book. I put all of myself into this body of work and pray that it blesses you. If it has made a difference in your life, there's a simple way to pay it forward. Just take a few minutes to share your testimony and point the way for others searching for the freedom you've found.

I appreciate it so much and promise to read your review!

# The Faster Way to Fat Loss After 40 Collective

How to Be Fit, Fabulous, and Fierce After 40

I know exactly how it feels when stubborn tummy, thigh, or arm fat just won't budge, or worse, keeps coming back, no matter how "clean" you eat or how much you exercise. After 40, your body changes, and those old rules of ***"eat less, move more"*** simply don't work. I've been there, and I've helped countless women just like you finally break the cycle.

That's why I created the Faster Way to Fat Loss After 40 Collective, an online support group that offers step-by-step guidance through the Faster Way program, plus accountability and support so you're never doing this alone.

Inside the Collective, you'll get:

- Weekly trainings to guide you through each step
- Weekly group coaching + accountability with me, Cynthia

- Private online chat for daily support and encouragement
- Guest speakers sharing tips and inspiration

Together, we'll melt stubborn fat, balance hormones, boost energy, sleep better, and help you finally feel confident, sexy, and strong, without worrying about it coming back.

This is a monthly online membership, join anytime, stay as long as you need, and return whenever you want a little boost.

You don't have to do this alone. I'm here, and so is your community.

*Learn More Here:* https://bit.ly/Over40Collective

# The Faster Way to Fat Loss After 40

## Companion Cookbook

If you're ready to take what you've learned in The Faster Way to Fat Loss After 40 and make it simple to follow day-to-day, I created something just for you.

**The Faster Way to Fat Loss After 40 Cookbook**

With this cookbook, you'll have **all of the recipes and meal plans in one easy-to-access place**—so you don't have to flip through pages or print anything out.

Inside, you'll find:

- A 7-day recipe plan and grocery list for your **liver detox**
- A **7-day parasite and candida cleanse** with recipes and guidance
- Simple meals for your **keto-style fat-burning phase**
- **Cycle-syncing recipes and meal plans** for perimenopause, menopause, and post menopause

Each section is designed to support **fat loss, hormone balance, energy, and overall wellness.** You'll also find meals tailored to your **menstrual or lunar cycle** to help you stay aligned with your body.

I created this cookbook so you can follow the program with ease—**no guesswork, no overwhelm,** just practical meals to support your journey.

**Get your copy here:**

https://amzn.to/3OH5kL7

or at

www.CynthiaRay.com

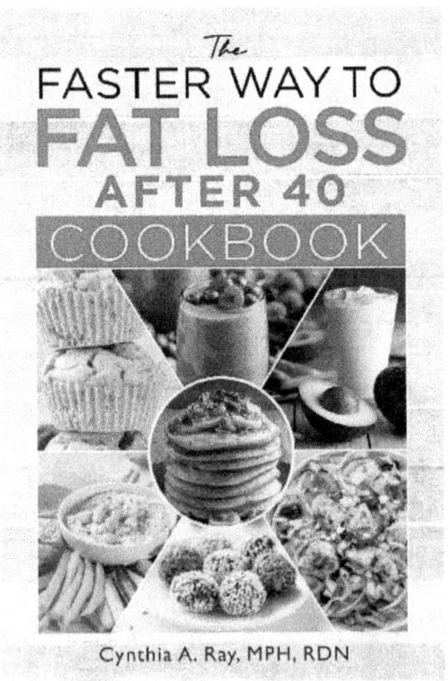